COUPLE SEXUAL AWARENESS

COUPLE SEXUAL AWARENESS

BARRY & EMILY MCCARTHY

CARROLL & GRAF PUBLISHERS, INC.
NEW YORK

Second Carroll & Graf paperback edition 1998

Carroll & Graf Publishers, Inc.
19 West 21st Street
New York, NY 10010

Library of Congress Cataloging-in-Publication Data available

ISBN: 0-7867-0525-6

Manufactured in the United States of America

Contents

COUPLE SEXUAL AWARENESS

I
ENHANCEMENT

1

IS THERE SEX AFTER MARRIAGE?

Sex comes naturally, there is one right way to have a successful marriage, being happily married is the norm, the more intimacy the better, and if you love each other and communicate, everything will be fine. Right? Wrong! Unrealistic expectations, especially about intimacy and sexuality, are a major source of marital frustration and unhappiness. Couples lack awareness and understanding of the complex processes involved in building a vital marital bond and maintaining satisfying marital sex.

This book is directed to couples who want a satisfying, stable marriage and fulfilling marital sexuality. You will learn concepts and techniques to enhance respect, trust, emotional intimacy, and sexual satisfaction. We focus on improving sexual communication and expression. Instead of dictating one right way, we believe each couple needs to develop their own marital and sexual style.

Sexuality is not the most important factor in marriage, but is integral to a successful marriage. The functions of sexuality are to serve as a shared pleasure, a means to deepen and reinforce intimacy, and a tension reducer to deal with the stresses of life and marriage. When sex goes well it contributes 15 to 20 percent to the marriage—energizing the marital bond and making it special. When sex is problematic, it drains positive feelings. In marriages where sex is dysfunctional or nonexistent it becomes 50 to 75 percent of the relationship, draining the marriage of intimacy and vitality.

We urge couples to avoid the happy-ever-after approach to marriage. We emphasize the importance of "couple time," the

3

need to commit psychological energy to ensure marital vitality and satisfaction. Marriage is an active, ongoing process, not a static asset you can take for granted.

SEXUALITY AND MARRIAGE

Cultural, parental, and peer pressure to marry abound. Over 90 percent of people marry. Among the almost 50 percent who divorce, the great majority remarry. Marriage is the most popular voluntary institution in America. But marital intimacy—like a freshly cut rose—blooms early and then fades into habit and routine. The concept of a genuinely intimate and sexually satisfying marriage draws disbelief, guffaws, and cynicism.

Sex books have been directed toward the young, with discussions of premarital sex, safer sex, "meaningful relationships," and finding the "right" person to marry. It appears sexuality begins at sixteen and ends at thirty, its prime purpose to get the person safely—without disease, an unwanted pregnancy, or destructive relationships—settled into marriage. The image is a movie—the couple marries and has totally satisfying intercourse with simultaneous orgasm. The assumption is they live happily ever after as "The End" flashes on the screen. Unfortunately—or rather fortunately—life, sex, and marriage are more real and complex than that.

We focus on the uniqueness and complexity of your marital and sexual bond. Sex does not exclusively belong to the young or newly married. You are a sexual person from the day you are born until the day you die. Sex in marriage constitutes the major portion of most people's sexual lives, yet has received surprisingly little scientific or public attention. Marital sexuality is a subject hidden behind self-defeating attitudes and myths.

WHO WE ARE AND WHY WE WROTE THIS BOOK

Through Barry's clinical practice in marital and sex therapy, conducting sexual enhancement workshops, teaching human sexuality, and thinking about our marriage, we have come to believe that several concepts are crucial. One is the importance of setting aside couple time and valuing intimacy; another is being aware of sensuality, which is the basis of sexual responsivity, and the

role of nondemand pleasuring; the importance of erotic stimulation and the freedom to let go and enjoy orgasm; and the need
to reduce performance anxiety and replace unrealistic expectations with a flexible, pleasure-oriented, broad-based view of marital sexuality. This book will offer strategies and techniques to
help you develop an intimate sexual relationship which enhances
marital satisfaction and stability.

We write from the dual perspective of Barry's clinical work
with couples and our personal involvement in the subject matter.
Barry is fifty-four and Emily fifty-two. We have been married
thirty-one years and have three children and one grandchild. This
is the seventh book (and our favorite) we've written together.
Couple Sexual Awareness integrates our views about the importance of intimacy, sexuality, and marriage. Throughout we offer
case material (names and details altered to protect confidential-
ity) as well as observations from our life—not as the "right"
path for you, but as concrete illustrations of how real couples
change and negotiate transitions in their marriage and sexual
relationship.

POSITIVE GUIDELINES

Your marital and sexual relationship will be more satisfying
if it is based on solid information, awareness, comfort, communication, and positive attitudes. Knowledge is power. Awareness and attitude change are necessary, but not sufficient. The
couple must change their manner of relating. Expectations must
be reassessed and communication skills improved. It is important
to understand and cope with the challenges of an ongoing marriage, adopt a pleasure-oriented rather than performance-oriented
view of sex, and increase the frequency and variety of
affectional, sensual, and sexual experiences. As attitudes and behavior change, feelings of closeness and intimacy grow.

We do *not* believe there is "one right way" to have a successful marriage. In fact, we feel just the opposite. Each individual and couple has a unique set of experiences, attitudes,
values, preferences, feelings, and life situation. Each couple can
develop a marital and sexual style that satisfies their needs, circumstances, and values.

It is amazing that couples who are knowledgeable and do well in other life areas can be so naive about intimacy. Barry sees couples who are financial wizards and sophisticated about "the good life," but whose marriages are essentially empty. Americans value marriage as an institution, but few are skilled at communicating feelings, building emotional intimacy, making sexual requests, reinforcing marital commitment, and enjoying intimate sexuality. The challenge is to integrate these guidelines and skills so you can build and maintain a satisfying and secure marriage.

WHAT IS YOUR MARITAL AND SEXUAL STYLE?

What do we mean by a marital and sexual style? By the time they've been married two years, a couple has established a pattern of roles and behaviors—for example, who gets up to make the coffee or who chooses the music they listen to. Their style of communication may be functional, but often is not. The couple talk, but their conversation is about sports, neighborhood events, finances, chores, or children's activities rather than sharing personal perceptions and feelings.

Research evidence demonstrates there are four viable marital styles:

1. Complementary couples—who maintain a balance of individuality and intimacy, acknowledge and validate each other's strengths and contributions, and value their marriage, although often undervalue the role of sexuality.
2. Conflict-minimizing couples—who organize their lives along traditional male-female roles, value stability and children, have clear domains of influence, and underplay strong emotions, including sexual feelings.
3. Best friend couples—who personify the cultural ideal and represent the model we base our marriage on, which however is not the right style for most marriages. This model involves the deepest emotional intimacy. The risk is to underplay individuality, which can result in disappointment and inhibited sexual desire if the best-friend style stymies individual or couple growth.
4. Emotionally expressive couples—who express a wide range of emotions, from anger to sexual passion. This is the most exciting style, but also the most unstable. Intimacy

is like an accordion, sometimes the partners are very close and sometimes they're very distant.

Of course, no couple has a "pure" style. You need to establish a marital style which meets your individual and couple needs. One wanting a conflict-minimizing style and the other an emotionally expressive style could spell disaster.

A crucial couple issue involves the degree of intimacy. Contrary to what "pop psychology" books and talk radio say, more is not necessarily better. The couple needs to establish a balance between individual autonomy and coupleness. Likewise, they need to establish a mutually comfortable degree of intimacy which allows for connection and facilitates sexual desire. Too much closeness or too little connection inhibits sexual desire.

The third issue in a couple's style involves touching, intercourse frequency, and the importance of sex in their lives. Some people view sex as central, others think of sex as peripheral. The paradox is that when sex goes well, it is a positive, integral component of the marriage, but not a major one. However, when sex is problematic, dysfunctional or nonexistent, it plays an inordinately powerful role. The sad truth is, bad sex has a more powerful negative role than good sex has a positive role in marital satisfaction.

Until thirty years ago, little research was done to increase sexual knowledge. Even the so-called experts—psychologists, physicians, ministers, marriage counselors, and teachers—were minimally helpful. Their advice was based on theoretical notions or common myths. With the breakthrough research of Masters and Johnson and other behavioral scientists, our understanding of marital and sexual functioning has increased dramatically. The more information you have, the better able you are to make reasoned, productive decisions.

Our culture is heavily influenced by myths of romantic love. Couples believe love is enough for happiness. Loving feelings are necessary, but not sufficient, for a good marriage. Romantic love, which idealizes the partner and relationship, needs to be replaced by a broad-based, mature, and stable sense of intimacy. This means acceptance of the real person and strengths and weaknesses of the marriage. Intimacy allows you to deal with problems and failures as well as enjoy loving feelings and sexual highs. An intimate bond energizes you to deal with the real and complex issues present in any marriage, including sexual issues.

Our behavior is influenced by the models, especially parental models, we've observed. Yet you don't learn to be a communicative sexually comfortable couple from your parents, who were influenced by their parents and the lack of information and antisexual attitudes of their culture. Parents are viewed as nonsexual by their children. They are seen as parents only, rather than as individuals and a sexual couple. An informal study conducted in Barry's Human Sexual Behavior course found only one in four college students could imagine their parents having intercourse and only one in twelve could imagine their grandparents being sexual.

In addition to the absence of a parental model for intimate sexuality, most couples lack a good model for marital communication. Children see parents talking about family/child issues or practical problems. Anger expression is extreme—either irrational, destructive, violent or nonexistent. Seldom do children witness their parents expressing emotional support or engaging in constructive disagreement and conflict resolution. And heaven forbid that parents touch or kiss where the children might see them. The best way to learn a behavior is through observation, but few people have experienced good models of marital communication or affection. This book presents positive models of emotional intimacy and sexual comfort.

COUPLE STRATEGIES AND TECHNIQUES

You can learn and grow by employing specific change strategies and techniques. The strategy that most influences our marriage is "couple time." This is time we set aside for the two of us, without children, to talk about individual and couple issues rather than practical matters. This time could be associated with sex—for instance, twenty minutes after intercourse—but usually is not. A couple might sit over a drink, go for a walk and talk, share something they are happy and excited about, or discuss how they have been getting along the past week. We encourage setting aside at least one period a week for couple time. Some couples do this three or four times a week. This time does not *just* happen, it's *planned* to happen. It is recognized as a priority, planned into and valued in your busy schedule.

One of the benefits of being in therapy is that it provides a structured time to talk as a couple. When therapy ends, Barry encourages the couple to preserve this time since it's already built into their schedules. Instead of an office visit and a fee they go to lunch, take a walk, or meet at home and make love. Emily believes our healthiest communication technique is walks two or three times a week during which we share feelings and perceptions, deal with issues, make plans, or just enjoy the beauty of nature.

Once a month, or every other month, set aside a day for you as a couple. Keeping a relationship fresh, close, and enjoyable is a continual process of sharing experiences, communicating feelings, and giving yourself time and permission to be intimate. It is necessary to have time away from jobs, children, the phone, and friends. This allows you to experiment with sexual techniques, learn a new sport or hobby, or just be together in a relaxed atmosphere. A prevalent, self-defeating myth is that marriages do not need time or attention to remain satisfying. If businessmen put as little time and energy into their businesses as couples put into their marital relationships, we would have a bankrupt country. With so little attention, it's amazing marriages do as well as they do!

For a satisfying marriage there are four things a couple needs to do:

1. Communicate with and support each other.
2. Deal with negative feelings and conflicts in a constructive manner.
3. Laugh, share interests, and enjoy each other.
4. Have a satisfying sexual relationship.

The more comfortable and skilled the couple is, the more satisfying their marriage will be. These four basic elements are not inborn traits, nor do they naturally develop, even if a loving relationship exists. They are learned skills that require awareness and effort. Like any skill, from playing tennis to cooking, once learned it needs to be practiced and refined.

Don't allow your marital or sexual relationship to become routine and stagnant. Marriage is a continual process of changing and growing. As the poet/philospher Kahlil Gibran wrote, "A love that is not always growing is dying." A key to successful marriage is a commitment to integrate individual and couple changes. The marital relationship is a *process*. It is changing not only at twenty-five, but at forty-five, and just as much at seventy-five. You never stop learning and growing as a person, as a couple, and in your sexuality.

COMMUNICATION AND EMOTIONAL SUPPORT

When we speak of communication and emotional support, we are referring to a series of component skills:
1. Empathic listening for both content and feelings.
2. "Checking out," especially for intentions.
3. Empathic responding.
4. Use of "I" communications.
5. Making requests, not demands.
6. "Going my way" skill of negotiation.
7. Reaching agreements both can live with.
8. Monitoring the agreement for successful implementation.

The first and foremost skill is listening to the spouse in a respectful, empathic manner, understanding both content *and* feelings. Because of different socialization males often attend to content and problem solving while ignoring feelings, whereas females frequently focus on feelings and attend less to content or problem resolution. This is a major factor in the communication gap couples complain about. Take time to listen to the spouse, trying to "take the role of the other," to understand the issue from her viewpoint. When you assume you are right and the spouse is wrong, you fail to understand feelings and perceptions. Instead, you are waiting for him to finish so you can make your point. To be a good communicator, you must first be an empathic listener.

The second component skill is "checking out." Be sure you understand what was said, the intention, the spouse's feelings, and what is being requested. Reacting defensively, as if you'd been attacked or demands had been made, puts you in a power struggle rather than on the same intimate team. If you feel pressured or hurt by his comments, checking it out allows you to determine whether that was the intent, you misunderstood the message, or it was expressed in a confusing way. It is particularly important to check out your partner's intentions—is she trying to be helpful and make a positive point or is she angry and undercutting? One way to check out is to say, "I feel put down by your comment; did you mean it as a put-down?" Checking out before responding makes it more likely that the response will be constructive rather than defensive or a counterattack.

The third component skill is empathic responding. State your feelings and requests, keeping in mind the other's perceptions and feelings. This is very different from disparaging the spouse, giving "yes, but" responses, or counterattacking. Share your perceptions and feelings and express them within the context of being intimate friends. Marital communication is based on a positive influence model. Communicate in a respectful, responsive manner. The goal of empathic responding is for the partner to know he was heard. Your response conveys your feelings, perceptions, and requests.

The fourth component skill involves using "I" communications. This means saying "I want to go to the movies today; are you up for it?" "I feel sensuous right now and would love a chest rub; are you interested?" "I think we need to talk about our finances," or "I want to go out to dinner tonight." Be clear, direct, and straightforward with your feelings and what you want. Be your own agent rather than reacting with what you think she wants you to say. This is very different from a couple communication pattern of "What do you want to do?" "I guess you want to have sex," or "I don't care; how do you want to handle it?" "I" communications are honest. Take responsibility for your feelings and behavior. This involves taking risks which make you vulnerable to disappointment, but it's worth it.

Make requests, not demands. The fifth component skill is learning to make clear, assertive requests. This replaces communication which is either passive and indirect or aggressively demanding. The major difference between a request and a demand is that a request gives the partner a choice. You may not get precisely what you requested, but you should choose to work with the spouse rather than intimidate or coerce him. A demand puts pressure on her to give you what you want when you want it or there will be consequences. It is the difference between saying, "I would like you to stroke my penis slowly" and "You better turn me on by playing with me, or you won't get any tonight." Sexual demands cause sexual dysfunction and resentment; sexual requests result in pleasurable sex and emotional intimacy.

Going my way? The sixth component skill is learning to generate alternatives and set the stage for negotiating agreements. When two people with separate needs and preferences relate intimately, they are open to negotiation. A crucial negotiation technique is to replace a "No" with "No, I am not willing to give you a thirty-minute back rub, but I would like to snuggle for a few minutes." Instead of "No, I have a headache," you say, "I have a headache, and would like a neck rub. Let's see how I feel; we might stop there, have sex, or I could give to you sexually." In place of saying no and cutting off communication, offer an alternative that is acceptable to you. The partner decides if he is open to engaging in this or not. People assume that if they cannot have what they want, when and how they want it, they are not loved. The reality is you do not usually get things exactly your way. Couples fall into the power struggle trap: "my" way versus "your" way rather than a couple style of communicating and negotiating—"our" way.

The seventh component skill is reaching worthwhile agreements. Agreements are very different from compromises. Always compromising is a common couple trap. In compromises, neither person gets what he/she wants; they go along with a compromise neither enjoys. For example, if one wants to go to a French restaurant and the other wants Chinese food, they compromise on standard American fare, which neither enjoys. At a minimum, a couple needs to reach agreements both can live with. Ideally, they would negotiate an agreement in which each gets something and feels good about their ability to work out issues.

Negotiation, where you clearly state your feelings and wants, listen to the partner's, and reach an agreement in which each person gets at least some of her needs met, is preferable to compromise where you do something neutral so neither feels he/she lost. In this brand of compromise, you both lose! Making requests and considering alternatives adds to the sense of caring. For example, he might want fellatio and she might want a sexual massage with body lotion. They compromise by having intercourse with the woman on top, which is not what either wanted.

An agreement involves the woman receiving a sexual massage with lotion and then reciprocating with a sexual massage which includes fellatio and integrates multiple stimulation during intercourse. You can reach satisfying agreements, and in so doing, become a more intimate couple.

Good intentions are not enough. The eighth skill is putting in place a mechanism to monitor the agreement to ensure successful implementation. Often, the mechanism is simple—meeting for ten minutes once a week to be sure each person is doing what he/she agreed to. Sometimes, it is quite complex—having a written agreement, carrying a notecard to check off whether you did what you agreed to, or setting up three to five subgoals so you eventually reach the resolution you want.

DEALING WITH NEGATIVE FEELINGS AND CONFLICTS

People believe arguing is the opposite of intimacy. That's a self-defeating myth. Intimate couples *can* and *do* have hurt, disappointed, angry feelings. It's important to express these. Some couples brag they never fight. Such relationships are built on an unrealistic premise that presents a strong risk of explosion, resulting in feelings of deep hurt and betrayal. Learning to express hurt or angry feelings in an honest and constructive manner is a vital skill. It isn't easy, but it is worthwhile.

In a healthy relationship both spouses feel they can be honest, open, and vulnerable. This includes feelings of love, caring, and respect as well as hurt, anger, and disappointment. You say, "I am feeling angry about our financial situation." This is very different from, "You are a failure, you'll never learn to handle money." You need to acknowledge feelings, objectively view the situation with the intention of problem solving, and avoid blaming or putting down the spouse.

Learning to argue well does not mean you fight over each matter or let the spouse know immediately about each feeling. It certainly doesn't mean physical abuse or psychological coercion. This is aggressive and inappropriate, just as the couple who never fights is inhibited and frightened of expressing negative feelings.

Learning to deal constructively with conflict includes four component skills:
1. Ability to express negative feelings.
2. Expressing feelings in a nondestructive way, without ''hitting below the belt.''
3. Requesting a specific change in the spouse's attitude or behavior. The intention is to engage in constructive problem solving.
4. Ability to identify problems which can be resolved, problems which can be reduced, and problems which must be accepted and coped with.

The first skill—clearly stating feelings—means saying, ''I am hurt and angry when you come home three hours late and don't call'' instead of ''I hate you, you're an inconsiderate bastard.'' It means saying specifically what you are feeling and what is causing you to feel that way. It does not mean calling the spouse names, blaming or attacking, or saying she always does this or that and is hopeless. It means trying to solve the problem, not getting your way or making him feel guilty. Good conflict resolution skills include staying on the specific issue and feelings instead of dredging up past feelings and incidents. Stay with the here and now. Don't refight past battles and throw in old hurts, the proverbial ''kitchen sink'' fights.

The second skill involves arguing in nondestructive ways. It means saying, ''I feel hurt, confused, and discouraged when you don't show me the consideration to call'' instead of ''You're irresponsible and manipulative just like your mother.'' One of the best things about an intimate relationship is you feel safe, trustful, and accepted for the person you are. You can reveal vulnerabilities, the sad or bad moments of your life, concerns and inadequacies, without fear that they will be used against you. In a destructive fight, this is what happens; your vulnerabilities and weaknesses are used as ammunition for an attack, leaving you feeling betrayed and angry. In retaliation, the spouse ''goes for the jugular.'' The argument degenerates into a destructive power struggle or, in the colloquial, ''a pissing match.'' The couple is no longer trying to achieve something, each spouse is fighting not to lose. The worst example of this degenerative fighting style is demonstrated in the classic movie *Who's Afraid of Virginia Woolf?* Destructive couple arguments can turn into physical abuse, especially if one or both have been drinking.

Focus on your feelings rather than castigating the spouse. Be honest in owning your feelings rather than blaming them on the partner. If, during an argument, one hits below the belt, the offended spouse should not immediately counterattack but say, "I felt you just gave a low blow; did you intend to do it?" Most of the time, the spouse was simply caught in the heat of the argument. When made aware, the spouse backs off. If the spouse is maliciously being hurtful, this argument can only be destructive. Call a time-out and leave the situation. After a cooling-off period, when both of you are willing to argue constructively rather than engaging in an out-of-control fight, return to the issue.

The best time to air negative feelings is not in the heat of the moment, but when you have time and privacy to talk and solve problems. An important guideline is not to have arguments after midnight—nothing constructive happens between then and six in the morning—or when one or both people have been drinking. In terms of sex, deal with sexual conflicts when you're clothed and not in bed. Sexual arguments when you're nude and lying down make you too vulnerable to destructive comments, defensiveness, and striking back.

People use arguments as a means of emotional catharsis, getting gripes off their chest. You feel better for a while, but frustrations and anger build because the situation has not changed. It is important to express feelings rather than build resentments. But just expressing feelings is not enough!

The third component is to request a change that will alter the problem situation and alleviate bad feelings. State your feeling clearly: "I am hurt because you did not pay attention to me last night." "I'm disappointed that after you said you'd try the side-by-side intercourse position, you stopped when it was awkward." "I am frustrated when we make plans to solve financial problems and don't follow through." "I am disappointed you forgot to attend our daughter's recital after you promised you'd be there." It is just as important to make a specific request for change: "When I say we need couple time, I want us to find a time we can talk or go out to dinner." "Each week we will go over the family budget." "You need to apologize to Sue yourself rather than my doing it for you. Why don't you do something special with her next week?" Statements like "You have to change your attitude," "You will never change," or "You do not care" are nonproductive. They do not bring the changes you want. Taking a problem-solving rather than blaming approach, making specific requests for change, and following through on behavior change plans alleviate distressing feelings and situations. The more pervasive and chronic the problem, the more detailed a plan you'll need. This includes an active monitoring process and establishing smaller goals to facilitate change.

Of the concepts and skills we write about, the constructive expression of negative feelings is the hardest to integrate in our marriage. Our arguments involve tears and hurt feelings, at least on occasion. We have a commitment, a strong one, to avoid insulting each other or making the partner feel guilty. A major difficulty is waiting too long to discuss the problem because we don't want to complain about a spouse we love, one who is attentive and considerate in most ways. Once the issue is aired and an agreement made, we find the conflict resolution process was worthwhile.

People hope and wish that all conflicts can be resolved. The truth is they can't, no matter what you hear on talk shows or read in "pop psychology" books. A difficult but crucial skill is differentiating between problems which are resolvable (perhaps one third), problems which can be significantly reduced (more than half), and problems which must be accepted and coped with (the hardest 10-15 percent).

We have chronic problem areas, especially regarding finances, which we are unable to satisfactorily resolve. On occasion, we need to air feelings about the problem so frustrations and resentments do not build. This is an area of ongoing dialogue rather than a resolvable problem.

LAUGHTER AND SHARING

Couples are not naturally compatible. They need to evolve an enjoyable, satisfying style of being together, learn to laugh and enjoy activities and share interests. Having two or three activities which both people genuinely enjoy is a solid base for the couple. This could include playing tennis, going to the movies, playing cards or board games, eating ethnic foods, being active in a community group, listening to jazz, dancing, decorating the house, going camping, gardening, participating in a church discussion group, golfing, reading poetry, going to car races, traveling, or entertaining. Not all activities can or should be joint. Having nonshared interests and activities is good for an individual and beneficial for the marriage. The husband having a night out bowling with friends or taking a class and the wife having a bridge game or being involved in a women's group enhance individuality. It's important to maintain a healthy balance of individual and couple activities.

Couples who shared experiences when first married find they've grown apart, each is involved in separate activities with separate friends. Individual interests, activities, and friends are fine, but not at the expense of being a couple. Activities you did fifteen years ago might no longer be enjoyable, although you still do them out of habit. It is possible to revitalize old interests and be open to new interests, such as Chinese cooking lessons or square dancing. Shared activities might include practical tasks—learning to wallpaper or finish furniture. At least one activity involves being playful, whether playing bridge, hiking, racquetball, going to musicals, or visiting exhibits. It's important to share pleasurable activities.

Being able to laugh and accept idiosyncrasies and foibles is necessary; every person has weaknesses and irritating behaviors. Accept that some things will not work the way you hoped, don't react with anger. For instance, if the couple tries a new dessert for a dinner party and it comes out absolutely awful, it's better to laugh rather than pretending everything is fine and embarrassing the guests and yourselves. The ability to laugh at yourselves is especially important in the sex area. Even couples who are very satisfied find 5 to 10 percent of their sexual experiences ungratifying. The sex might be mediocre, boring, or a downright "bomb." Overreacting and becoming dejected or frustrated makes the problem worse. The couple who laughs and says, "tonight is just not our night for sex," will continue to have a vital sexual life.

A SATISFYING SEXUAL RELATIONSHIP

This leads us to our final skill area—building and maintaining an intimate, satisfying sexual relationship. Sex is not the central ingredient in marriage, but sexuality is integral to the marital bond. Sex serves as a reinforcer and energizer. When the couple's sex life is dysfunctional or nonexistent, it depresses and negates other aspects of the marriage. A lack of regular, fulfilling experiences creates a void. Sexual problems drain a marriage of intimacy and positive feelings. There are times in every marriage when life is dull, stressful, or unsatisfactory. During those times, sharing intimacy and sexuality helps you through.

There are three core elements to a satisfying sexual relationship:

1. Feelings of intimacy.
2. Comfort with nondemand pleasuring.
3. Erotic sexual scenarios and techniques (including intercourse and orgasm).

Sex is a natural physiological function, like breathing and eating, but satisfying sexual expression is learned. We have devoted an entire book, *Sexual Awareness*, to specific exercises to facilitate sexual communication and functioning. The principal skills are the ability to enjoy sensuous, nondemand pleasuring; making sexual requests, guiding the spouse in how to touch and stimulate you; learning to accept and follow the partner's guidance; being open to a range of sensual and sexual techniques; use of erotic stimulation, including fantasizing, to build arousal; enjoying erotic scenarios; saying no and requesting alternative pleasuring techniques; multiple stimulation before and during intercourse; using focused, rapid, rhythmic thrusting as you approach orgasm; letting go and being orgasmic; having intimate, bonding afterplay; and learning to laugh or shrug off unsatisfactory sexual experiences. In short, put pleasure and intimacy into your sexual life rather than seeing sex as a goal-oriented performance. The essence of sexuality is giving and receiving pleasure within the context of an intimate relationship.

One of the most prevalent myths is that marital sex becomes less frequent and enjoyable because you have learned all you can and tried everything there is to try. No matter how often you have sex, you can never experience all the variations and complexities of being with someone you love. In a truly creative, intimate relationship your desires, feelings, and awareness continue to evolve. As you age, you have different feelings and responses. The couple who falls into a dull, mechanical sexual relationship has no one to blame but themselves. Sexuality can and should be a positive force in marriage. Enjoy a pleasurable, intimate, quality sexual relationship, instead of focusing on performance and quantity. Youthful emphasis on frequency and performance are replaced by middle-years emphasis on quality, pleasure, and satisfaction. Couples in their twenties would benefit from developing creative, pleasure-oriented scenarios and techniques. This inoculates them against sexual problems as they age.

Some people, including our editor, wondered why we chose to focus on sexual intimacy as compared to other aspects of marriage. Traditionally, marital sex has been ignored and viewed as an unglamorous topic. Yet sexuality plays an integral, energizing role in marriage. When being sexual, couples are most open and intimate, one of the special experiences that makes being married worthwhile. With the growing awareness that divorce has more repercussions on individuals, children, and society than originally believed, and with the fear of HIV/AIDS, couples are motivated to make their marriages viable and vital. Intimacy and sexuality are crucial components in a satisfying, stable marriage.

The greatest need for marriages, including our own, is the consistent expenditure of time and psychological energy. Sexuality is more than genitals, intercourse, and orgasm. It includes the walks you take, affection inside and outside the bedroom, nondemand pleasuring, discussing intimate feelings while clothed, sharing feelings before and after intercourse. Sexuality is, verbally and physically, genitally and nongenitally, an expression of intimacy. Sexuality energizes the marital bond and promotes satisfaction and stability.

THE FOCUS OF THIS BOOK

This book is *not* intended to replace professional sex therapy. The focus is on increasing marital and sexual functioning by presenting guidelines for improving communication, constructively dealing with conflicts, negotiating change agreements, learning to laugh and enjoy couple activities, and promoting pleasurable and satisfying sexuality. For couples with a sexual dysfunction or dissatisfaction—50 percent of marriages—we present guidelines to resolve problems.

Individual chapters examine the marital bond, sexual variations, sex education for children, the transition to being a couple again, and being sexual after sixty. Additionally, we explore problem areas such as inhibited sexual desire, sexual dysfunction, healing from sexual trauma, extramarital affairs, dealing with illness, second marriage, and the mundane stresses of day-to-day living. A critical concept is the husband-wife bond as the primary relationship in a family.

We emphasize four themes—communication and support, expressing negative feelings constructively, laughing and enjoying each other, and developing and maintaining an intimate sexual bond. The prime focus is on intimacy and sexuality, but these attitudes and skills are relevant to other aspects of the marriage.

This manuscript is not like a novel in which you have to read each chapter in turn. Although there are continuities among chapters, each is self-contained with its own theme. Read those that are of immediate import to you. Some chapters could be read alone, others with your spouse; you might even read aloud to each other. However, reading is not enough—you need to discuss the concepts and guidelines and integrate them into your lives and marriage. This book could be read for information and attitude change, but will have maximum value if it involves interactive learning, helping you implement strategies and techniques to enhance your relationship.

Sexuality is an integral component of the marital bond. Satisfying sex promotes intimacy, shared pleasure, tension reduction, and energizes the bond between you and your spouse. Marriage requires the continued investment of psychological time and energy. Contrary to popular myth, couples report increased sexual quality and satisfaction over time. Middle-years couples are less athletic sexual performers, but can be intimate, high-quality lovers.

Couples sometimes become aware of dissatisfaction or problems as a result of reading or discussing issues. Marital and sex therapy are valuable in helping you work through communication difficulties and untangling problem areas. Some people are averse to the idea of counseling or therapy, seeing it as a sign of personal weakness, craziness, or their marriage being in big trouble. The contrary is true; seeking professional help is a sign of strength. You admit problems, work together to alleviate sources of stress, and consult a professional who can facilitate communication and problem solving. Appendix I discusses how to choose a marital or sex therapist.

Awareness and respect for the uniqueness of each couple is the basis of our approach. We hope our concepts and guidelines will encourage you to attend to your relationship and help you develop a satisfying marital and sexual style.

2
THE MARITAL BOND—RESPECT, TRUST, AND INTIMACY

Sexuality is a positive, integral part of your marital bond, but *not* the most important factor. This chapter will focus on core dimensions of the marital bond—respect, trust, and intimacy.

In books about marriage, communication is given prime billing—especially communicating feelings. Many experts believe empathic, clear, and direct communication guarantees a successful marriage. Communicating feelings is widely believed to be the principal element in happy marriages.

We stress the importance of communication, but it is *not* the prime element of a successful marriage. Unless there is equity in power, the communication process can become a sham. Unless respect, trust, and intimacy is the basis of your relationship, communication techniques will not be helpful.

Some couples play a communication game in which they pretend to communicate about a problem when, in fact, one partner has already determined how he or she wants it resolved and uses power to coerce the decision. An example might clarify this.

Carol and Tim

Carol and Tim's marriage was characterized by friends as open, sharing, and communicative. They talked about their feelings regarding all of their decisions. However, when the chips were down, the decision made was almost always what Tim decided it should be. Although Tim listened to and understood Carol's feelings and concerns, it was only logical to do it his way since he had the heavier schedule, made more money, and could not change appointments. Besides, he rationalized, Carol was overly emotional and sensitive.

The basis of the marital bond is respect for each other, trust that the partner has your best interests in mind and will not subvert agreements or intentionally hurt you, and being open, vulnerable, and emotionally intimate. Within this framework, the principles of open, clear, and direct communication are of great value. These same communication techniques in the context of a nontrusting relationship with a gross power imbalance are destructive. The communication process is a sham in a relationship like Carol and Tim's. For communication to be worthwhile there needs to be equity in power, self-respect, respect for the spouse, and a trusting relationship. Otherwise, communication techniques can be used in a manipulative or coercive manner.

RESPECT, TRUST, AND INTIMACY

These concepts are interrelated, but we will examine each separately and then discuss how they can be integrated in a marriage. The basis of marriage is a respectful, trusting friendship where emotional and sexual intimacy generate special feelings.

Respect. Respecting the spouse and accepting his/her strengths and weaknesses is the basis for a mature, intimate relationship. Knowing, understanding, and accepting the partner, which is the basis of respect, clashes with the cultural stereotype of romantic love. Respect emanates from a clear view of the spouse. It is not based on an emotional, rose-tinted perspective that ignores problematic behavior or difficult personality characteristics. Romantic love idealizes the partner, respect entails knowing the spouse's positive and negative traits while still respecting and loving him.

Respecting the spouse does not mean you have to agree with everything she does, nor does it mean there will be no individual growth or change. Marriage works best when based on a positive influence model of change.

Respect includes not demeaning the spouse, especially in front of children or friends. It encompasses supporting the spouse, seeing him as your intimate friend as opposed to a critic or competitor. When she is experiencing a serious problem at work or with the children, is phobic or depressed, he is empathic and supportive, not blaming or condescending. Be aware of and emphasize the partner's strengths and avoid dwelling on failings. People love us for our strengths; the spouse loves and respects you for your strengths and weaknesses. For example, Barry acts like a fish out of water when it comes to repairing equipment around the house and Emily nearly hyperventilates if she has to entertain more than four people. We acknowledge problem areas without losing respect for each other. When there is a difficulty that needs to be dealt with and changed—Barry not monitoring his diabetes or Emily ignoring financial responsibilities—the issue is confronted in a problem-solving, nonpunitive way. We do not engage in put-downs. Maintaining an equitable balance of power is crucial to self-respect and respect for the spouse.

Trust. Talk of respect turns couples off. They fear love and romance have been taken out of the relationship and replaced by a realistic, functional partnership with little emotion. Respect is a necessary, but certainly not sufficient, basis for a satisfying and secure marriage. Trust and intimacy are vital.

Trust integrates pragmatic and emotional components. Marriage is a functional relationship between two people, but to be satisfying it must be more than that. Trust that the spouse cares about you and has your best interests at heart is crucial. Trust involves maturity and caring about the partner, as well as his caring for you. A trusting relationship means believing the spouse would not intentionally hurt you or subvert your needs.

Trust in the spouse and his intentions is the emotional basis for a satisfying marriage. Couples under stress or in a crisis will successfully hold their ground as long as trust in their ''coupleness'' remains intact. Once trust has been breached, it is difficult, although not impossible, to regain. All couples experience stress, negative feelings, anger, disappointment, and conflict of needs. If the sense of trust is maintained, they can deal with problems and emerge a stronger couple, having learned from and survived the stressful situation.

Intimacy. Emotional intimacy is the focus of this chapter, although both emotional and sexual intimacy are vital for marital satisfaction. Emotional intimacy nurtures the marital bond. A chief ingredient in intimacy is freely and comfortably disclosing feelings, thoughts, and perceptions. This means revealing positive and negative feelings. Our preferred model of marriage is one in which the partners view each other as intimate friends where secrets, perceptions, feelings, hopes, and problems are shared. Some couples prefer greater emotional autonomy, which is fine as long as it is agreeable to both. A new myth is you can never have too much intimacy. You need to retain individuality; intimacy does not mean total enmeshment and giving up one's sense of self. Trouble arises when one demands intimacy and the other demands autonomy. The pursuer-distancer dynamic puts stress on the marital bond. The couple needs to establish a mutually comfortable level of emotional intimacy.

Intimacy includes a comfortable way of being together. Some couples enjoy talking about feelings and aspirations. Other couples do best when talking is combined with an activity like walking, playing board games, going to dinner, working on a household chore, attending a concert or playing golf. Being a couple includes, but is certainly not limited to, discussing feelings; integrating talking and touching is an important ingredient in intimacy.

Being there for each other in difficult and sad times is integral to intimacy. To paraphrase Kahlil Gibran, there are many people you can laugh with but you especially value people you can cry with. In an intimate marriage you celebrate happy moments as well as acknowledge you have survived painful or traumatic experiences. Being there during tough times makes the bond of trust and intimacy stronger.

Tonia and Roger

Tonia and Roger recently completed a couples' communication workshop. It was a high-quality, professionally organized training where they learned effective listening techniques—eye contact, nonverbal attending, verbally validating, reflecting feelings. Yet they continued to have draining arguments, and marital dissatisfaction increased. Their minister referred the couple to Barry for marital therapy.

After three assessment sessions it was clear intimacy and communication were not the problem. The therapeutic focus was their marital agreements and how they decided, or more to the point didn't decide, who did what in the relationship. Tonia worked three-quarters-time as a secretary. She had almost full responsibility for Jill, their eleven-year-old daughter, as well as full responsibility for the house. Family and social activities were organized by Tonia. Roger was quite unhappy with his job as an inspector for the building department. This dissatisfaction dominated his life. He complained incessantly about money and work. Roger spent Sunday afternoons drinking beer and watching sports on TV.

Roger and Tonia loved each other and communicated about a variety of issues, including parenting, couple friendships, and relationships with extended family. But *love* is *not* enough to sustain a marriage. Couples have to respect each other and be able to talk about and resolve stresses and problems.

The topic they studiously avoided was Tonia's lack of respect for the way Roger handled frustration with his job. She understood and empathized with his feelings, but disliked how he dealt with them—he was acting like a macho teenager. When the issue was confronted, Roger was evasive. He was not proud of his passivity regarding the job situation. However, Roger maintained that since it was as it was and his job brought in a good deal more money than Tonia, she had no right to hassle him about how he spent his time and handled frustrations.

Feeling a surge of power, Tonia began making demands of Roger. He felt she was pushing him around, and became defensive and resentful. This could easily have degenerated into a bitter power struggle that would have threatened marital trust. Marriages work best when based on a positive influence process, which promotes respect and trust and is a solid basis from which to address and resolve problems. It is preferable to confront a difficult issue in a respectful, problem-solving manner.

A further complication, which intrudes on many marriages, was that each spouse talked to same-sex friends and family who supported his/her viewpoint. Roger's male friends assured him that women hassled husbands and want them to be "good little boys." The only way to deal with women was to show them who was boss—to ignore them. Tonia's friends told her men were unreliable and wanted to be "playboys." The way to make your point was to threaten to leave or withhold sex. With friends like this, you don't need enemies. Unfortunately, friends and family take sides and make judgments that exacerbate marital difficulties, sabotaging the conflict resolution process.

Barry encouraged Tonia to use her communication skills to make clear and direct requests. Tonia needed to stop making demands, issuing ultimatums, and disparaging Roger. Roger was urged to listen to her requests and take a hard, objective look at his attitudes and behavior. His job frustrations were real but he allowed them to dominate their lives. Roger resolved to resume control of his life and made a commitment either to change his job within the department or, failing that, to seek another job. Realistically, it would take at least six months to engineer a satisfactory job change. During this period he resolved not to use job frustration as a way to avoid marital and parental involvement. Specifically, Roger agreed to limit his drinking/sporting with male friends to once a week and consult Tonia before making plans.

Roger had ignored responsibilities to Tonia, Jill, and the house. He resumed those responsibilities, and Tonia was surprised by her reluctance to give them up even though intellectually that was what she wanted. This is not unusual—it's hard to give up power and prerogatives, whether you're a woman or a man.

Once the power balance and mutual respect returned, the same communication techniques that had not helped three months before became useful. Roger and Tonia experienced renewed emotional and sexual intimacy. Most important, they had a commitment to problem solving and reaching mutually acceptable agreements.

Power. The women's movement has made us aware of power issues in relationships. The traditional model, in which the man is in control of household, financial, and family decisions because he earns more money, with the wife as handmaiden in charge of cleaning, cooking, and children, was never valid. Men believed money equaled power. Since traditionally men made more money, they did not have to share in less pleasant tasks such as housecleaning, changing diapers, and driving children's car pools. Our culture puts too much emphasis on money and power, but this *definitely should not* be so in marriage.

A joke among therapists is that the most difficult couple to treat are two lawyers overconcerned with protecting their bargaining position and not showing weakness. Techniques that may be effective in the business world are harmful in intimate relationships. Power plays and intimidation are counterproductive in marriage. You get what you want in a specific situation, but in the long run it's costly for the relationship. Resentment and desire to retaliate are destructive to the marital bond. Power manipulation allows you to win a battle, but you lose the war for a trusting, intimate marriage.

Couples report greater satisfaction when there is an equitable sharing of power. Each spouse has domains in which he/she takes initiative and is dominant. Because a spouse accepts the partner's initiative does not mean he is powerless. Power is not something that is shared fifty-fifty on each issue. Equal power in all areas is an unrealistic expectation and an unworkable model. Feeling comfortable with your sense of power and being aware of the spouse's domain facilitates an equitable balance of power which allows respect, trust, and intimacy—including sexual expression—to grow.

COMMUNICATION

Good communication facilitates marital functioning. In the first chapter we discussed these communication skills:

1. Emphatic listening for both content and feelings.
2. "Checking out," especially for intentions.
3. Empathic responding.
4. Use of "I" communications.
5. Making requests, not demands.
6. "Going my way" skill of negotiation.
7. Reaching agreements both can live with.
8. Monitoring the agreement for successful implementation.

Rather than repeating ourselves, we will focus on communication exercises. Marital communication is an ongoing process based on the assumption that each person's needs and feelings matter. You trust the spouse is negotiating in good faith rather than engaging in a power play or placating you. The agreements are not empty promises, they result in behavioral follow-through.

Jenny and Tom

Jenny and Tom had been married twenty-two years and were able to deal with most aspects of their relationship, except for one persistent problem. At issue was the amount of time Jenny spent on the phone talking to friends. This had been a sore point for over twenty years. It was so conflictual, they avoided talking about it, since it always ended in a replay of the same shouting, accusatory fight. The problem wouldn't go away. When Tom came home in a bad mood or wanted to talk to Jenny and found her on the phone, he'd make a snide comment and a cold war began that could last for days.

In communicating about a chronic, difficult problem, a crucial guideline is to approach it anew with a commitment to stay focused on the present and refuse to refight old battles. One suggestion is to use an outside person—someone you like, trust, and is willing to do it—as an objective resource to keep you on task. Tom and Jenny had the discussion with the help of a mutual friend whose profession was labor relations negotiator.

The format gave each time to speak. The partner's role was to empathically listen for both feelings and content, in a respectful and caring manner, without being distracted by what to say next, or getting ready to make a point. Then the roles were reversed. The partners took their time in going through the process conscientiously instead of rushing to solve the problem.

Jenny wanted Tom to understand how much she enjoyed talking with friends. This was not a reflection on him, although she also wanted Tom to listen to her, especially when she talked about shared worries. Tom felt rejected, hurt, and angry, believing she cared more for friends and the telephone than for him. Both agreed this was a serious problem. Each wanted the other to change.

For the first time each saw the emotional and content issues clearly. They did not get off task by refighting battles and bringing up old hurts. This format made it possible to look at alternatives and negotiate an agreement. Jenny agreed to talk with friends no more than half an hour when Tom was in the house. If she was on the phone when Tom came in, she'd break off the conversation within five minutes. If need be, she could call the person back. Tom agreed to spend time listening to Jenny's feelings and concerns. He no longer perceived her phone conversations as a personal rejection. In making this agreement, they felt validated even though neither got exactly what he wanted. They agreed to treat a problematic incident as a lapse, not a negation of the agreement or a reason to start the battle again. This is crucial. Even when you communicate clearly and come to an agreement, it does not mean the problem will never again rear its ugly head. Problems and irritations occur in the most solid marriage, even when the partners have the best of intentions. Hopefully, when the issue comes up again, they're better prepared to handle it. The best response is to reinstate the previous agreement and act accordingly.

Marital communication is an ongoing process. You can't rest on your laurels. There are no perfect people and no perfect marriages. Don't blithely say, ''We communicate about in-laws,'' or ''We communicate about money,'' and leave it at that. As parents age, new issues arise. In this era of competition and economic change you have to communicate *regularly* about money matters. We suggest the following exercises to facilitate the communication process. These techniques were developed in marital therapy. We've found them of value in our marriage.

Exercise One: Sharing. Once a week for a month set aside at least one hour where you have privacy and no distractions. Turn off the TV and put on the answering machine (or take the phone off the hook). You have one agenda—to share something about yourself and discuss feelings. No problem solving, no financial or parenting decisions, no talk about neighborhood or politics— the agenda is you, the spouse, and individual and couple perceptions and feelings. We suggest the following format:

1. State perceptions and feelings clearly and directly, using ''I'' language.
2. Before the spouse responds, she summarizes what she heard. Be sure she understands your perceptions and feelings.
3. She states her perceptions and feelings clearly and directly, using ''I'' language.
4. Again, be sure her perceptions and feelings are understood.

The couple's initial reaction is to find this too mechanistic. This technique forces you to slow down the communication process, really listen to the spouse and respond empathically (defensiveness or counterattacking is not appropriate). Put yourself in the role of the other. This feels awkward initially, but as you become comfortable and refine communication skills, you can use these techniques with greater flexibility. It's a bit like learning tennis; at first it's formal and structured, but once you learn the basics, you can adapt it to your game—in this case, your couple communication style.

Exercise Two: Disclosing a secret. Set aside at least an hour of couple time. Think of an experience or secret you have not shared with the spouse. The secret you choose need not be dramatic. It can be an experience, attitude, dream, or feeling. The secret could be feelings about your first date, a disturbing fantasy or dream, an embarrassing childhood experience, the first time you ever did something entirely on your own, an incident where you felt humiliated or ashamed.

State your motivation for sharing this secret and what you want from the spouse. The reason for this is to reassure the spouse, as well as to remind yourself, that your intention is not hostile or a way of "getting" the spouse under the guise of openness and honesty. Do you want feedback, suggestions, or simple acceptance? Some people prefer to disclose the secret at the beginning, others want to discuss the context, motivations, and feelings before sharing the secret. Whichever way you prefer is fine—as long as you do it.

Once shared, don't let the disclosure drop. Discuss how she feels about your secret. Stay with the feelings it evokes; don't analyze the partner's reaction as a way of diverting your focus. People who guard secrets from everyone, including the spouse and best friends, do not feel fully accepted. You tell yourself that if someone knew the secret they would think less of you or reject you. A well-known clinical adage is "You're only as sick as your secrets." You need to accept yourself with your disappointments, traumas, and embarrassments. You want to feel understood and respected by those close to you, especially the spouse. Don't switch to discussing the partner's secret until you've fully discussed yours. Allow a few days to lapse before discussing the spouse's secret.

Once you've had the experience of sharing a secret, it is easier to discuss feelings about other sensitive topics in a less formal manner. It gives you permission to share a difficult secret—childhood abuse, fears or experiences of failure, having been fired, being sexually humiliated.

Exercise Three: Your parents' marriage as a model. Parents are a major influence. They determine what you learn about marriage from observing them and their marital communication. People associate therapy with the stereotype of the "shrink" who analyzes childhood feelings and discovers the parents as the root cause of all problems. Actually, therapists no longer make childhood memories their primary focus, and we strongly recommend against doing this in your marriage. We do not agree with therapists or popular writers who engage in "mother bashing" or "father bashing." This exercise goes in a very different direction—its focus is on increasing awareness and understanding of your parents and their marriage.

In discussing your parents' marriage, first highlight aspects you admire and would like to incorporate into your marriage. Then pinpoint aspects you view as unsuccessful or inappropriate. Consider these as psychological traps to be aware of and monitor. These areas must be approached with careful thought and planning so your life and marriage function differently. Don't repeat destructive patterns.

It's difficult to be objective about parents; there is a tendency to be emotional/subjective—overly positive or totally negative. Try to be as specific as possible about both strengths and weaknesses. It is valuable to hear the spouse's perceptions of your parents' marriage, especially if the spouse is objective and specific. You do not have to agree with the spouse—after all, they're your parents—but her perceptions can broaden your perspective.

Don't throw the spouse's disclosure about his traps back at him during a fight. One of the advantages of an intimate marriage is that you can share concerns and vulnerabilities without fear of being humiliated or taken advantage of. How has your parents' model influenced your marriage? You are an adult, responsible for your life and marriage. Accept that responsibility—don't blame parents. This exercise can help you see them as people with strengths and weaknesses. Perhaps it will even help you deal more effectively with your aging parents.

Exercise Four: Expressing negative feelings and requesting specific changes. The idea of scheduling an argument is a far cry from traditional marital advice. Frustrations, disappointments, and conflicts exist in all intimate relationships. A crucial couple strategy is to communicate hurt or angry feelings and request changes before those feelings blow up into a major, destructive fight, or worse, a chronic problem. Don't allow yourselves to be stuck in the cycle of blame-defensiveness, attack-counterattack. Most couples do not feel right about proceeding in this rational, problem-solving manner. They see it as natural to have unplanned, explosive, destructive fights. Expressions of hurt and frustration are normal in a relationship; name calling, vindictive fights are not.

One partner takes the initiative and brings up an issue she is hurt or disappointed about. Don't blame the spouse for these feelings. They're your feelings, take responsibility for them. Use "I" language ("I feel hurt") not "you" language ("You're to blame for hurting me"). Pick one issue and stay with it. Once the partner understands your feelings and perceptions, make a clear, specific request for change. Remember, it's a request, not a demand. The spouse can decide whether to accept your request or offer an alternative to address the problem.

Be sure this issue is aired and a change negotiated before going on to the spouse's feelings and request for change. The spouse's feelings/request should be dealt with at a separate time and treated as a separate issue. This reduces the possibility of a counterattack on the same or a closely related issue. Stay away from tit-for-tat agreements, they lead to paralysis and resentment. The purpose of stating feelings and requesting a change is not to overpower, intimidate, or embarrass the spouse. Conflict resolution is not a competitive game with a winner and a loser. When you learn to share feelings, make requests, discuss alternatives, negotiate changes, reach mutually acceptable agreements, and follow through with a change plan, your marriage is the winner.

Exercise Five: Acknowledging strengths and accepting compliments. For many couples, this is the most difficult exercise. We say we want compliments, we need pats on the back. We are disappointed and bitter when we don't receive a "thank you" or a kiss to acknowledge the good and caring things we do. Yet we have a hard time genuinely stating strengths and positive characteristics as well as listening to and accepting compliments, especially from the spouse. We suggest that the wife go first because in our culture women have been discouraged from being complimentary about themselves and acknowledging strengths. Little girls are told to be quiet and proper, not verbal and vain.

Set a timer for three minutes. You have three minutes to talk about positive aspects of yourself and your strengths, with the spouse listening attentively. Say positive things without qualifications. Give yourself permission to say, "I am proud of the way I planned and built the patio," not "I did okay but it wasn't as good as the Jones's professional job." State what you respect and like about yourself. Look at the spouse as you speak, without being embarrassed or apologetic for "bragging on yourself." Three minutes is a short period of time, but some people feel it's an eternity when the task is self-acknowledgment. You owe yourself at least three minutes to acknowledge positive characteristics, strengths, and achievements.

When you've completed this, the spouse has three minutes to say what he respects and values about you. He can reinforce what you've said, but it's especially worthwhile if he chooses strengths and positive attributes you did not mention or downplayed. Don't be afraid to mention points that seem small; the only guideline is the feelings and statements must be genuine.

You could change roles during this exercise or wait a day to reverse roles. Be honest; don't try to compete by saying more things or giving just the right compliment. After you've completed the exercise, spend time discussing how you felt about giving and receiving positive feedback. It will become easier to give and receive compliments and acknowledge aspects of yourself, the spouse, and marital bond that you value.

CLOSING THOUGHTS

These exercises are designed in a structured, formal manner. Ongoing communication is not structured or formal. We suggest you continue to share feelings, discuss difficult issues, talk about family of origin and extended family relationships, confront hurt or angry feelings and request changes, and give compliments and acknowledge positive attributes. Communicating comfortably permits you to feel secure and satisfied with yourself as a person and the marital relationship.

For a stable and satisfying marital bond, there needs to be a sense of equity, as well as clear, comfortable, and genuine communication. As with sexual aspects of the relationship, once you've achieved this balance, you cannot rest on your laurels. You change as people and your marriage changes. Devote time and psychological energy to reinforce the marital bond of respect, trust, and intimacy.

3
NONDEMAND PLEASURING

The line between affection and sex is very clear. Affection is something you do with clothes on, involves kissing, hand-holding, and/or hugging, and can be done in public. Traditionally, affection was viewed as the woman's domain. Sex involves nudity, intercourse, and orgasm. Traditionally, sex was the man's domain. Affection and sex have been viewed as altogether different and separate activities. This rigid dichotomy subverts marital intimacy and sexuality while reinforcing traditional, self-defeating, double-standard sexual socialization.

The concept of nondemand pleasuring introduces an entirely different way of conceptualizing and experiencing affection, sensuality, eroticism, and sexuality. It challenges the traditional arbitrary distinctions. Most importantly, nondemand pleasuring discards the view that women and men are different in their emotional and physical need for touch. Pleasuring does away with the dichotomy between affection and sex, viewing touch as a continuum from hand-holding to intercourse. Touching can occur inside and outside the bedroom, may be initiated by the man or woman, can be clothed, semi-clothed, or nude. It meets needs of both people for physical and emotional connection.

Integral to the touching/pleasuring continuum is the concept of sensuality. Sensuality is done in private, includes some degree of nudity, involves experiences like bathing or showering together, back rubs, body caresses, and slow, tender, exploratory, caring touching. Sensuality includes both nongenital and genital touching. Sensuality is pleasure-oriented, not orgasm-oriented.

Sexuality is more than genitals intercourse, and orgasm. We

are unequivocally in favor of intercourse and orgasm, which are integral to sexual satisfaction. However, when you limit sex to intercourse you cheat yourself and the marriage of a range of affectionate, sensual, and erotic experiences. Affection, sensuality, and nondemand pleasuring provide the basis for intimacy and sexual desire. The essence of sexuality is giving and receiving pleasurable touch.

Couples who value nondemand pleasuring report increased closeness and touching, with increased arousal, intercourse and orgasm too. There are many ways to express intimate feelings and many bridges to sexual desire. Many women avoid engaging in extended, sensual kissing unless they are prepared to proceed to intercourse. If she felt free to kiss in a sensual manner, for its own sake, to elicit desire for a later time, or see if kissing results in arousal, there would be more opportunities to share sensuality and sexuality. The husband caresses the spouse's breast or she touches his penis with a sense of playfulness and openness which increases the exchange of pleasure and opportunities for eroticism. If breast and penis touch is restricted only to foreplay leading to intercourse, there will be fewer playful times and less intercourse. Nondemand pleasuring, which includes affection and sensuality, is integral to the relationship, not restricted to the bedroom before intercourse. Couples who have only two gears—the first a ritual kiss in the morning and at night while the other is intercourse and orgasm—miss opportunities to share intimacy, pleasure, and eroticism.

Touching is an excellent example of how the premarital attitudes and experiences of women and men interfere with marital sexuality. If touching is to strengthen the marital bond, the wife and husband have to overcome their adolescent misconceptions and enjoy a range of nongenital and genital pleasuring. Affection, pleasuring, eroticism, and intercourse are valued by both people.

Jan and Craig

As an adolescent Craig both loved and hated petting games. He loved the sense of adventure and conquest when he'd "get farther," but was frustrated that the woman held power and would not let him have "the real thing." He swore that once

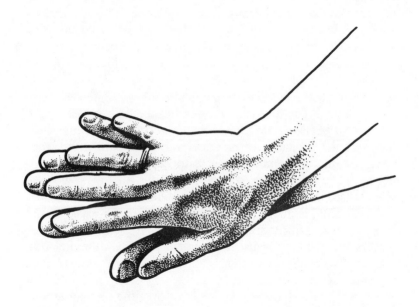

The basis of nondemand pleasuring is comfort with touching. Put your hand upon his and show him how and where you like being touched.

married he would never play those games again. Jan had a very different perception of touching and quite different experiences. She enjoyed the romanticism and sense of play that accompanied kissing, caressing, and stroking. However, she felt pushed and imposed on by men wanting more breast and genital stimulation, and tired of defending herself against the accusation of being a "tease." Instead of enjoying touching and arousal, she learned to experience the male's erection as sexual pressure for intercourse, or at least for bringing him to orgasm. This was not nondemand pleasuring, his erection was a demand. She hated the pressure of having to say "no" and pushing the man away. What could have been a pleasurable experience turned into a power struggle.

Jan and Craig met during their junior year in college, when they were dating other people. Both were aware of an attraction, but since each was involved with someone else, they developed a friendship. When they returned to school the following year, Jan learned Craig was no longer dating the same woman. They met for coffee, and Jan remembers feeling strongly attracted and a special sensation when Craig touched her arm. As they left the café, he took her hand and went for a walk in the woods surrounding the campus. Their first kiss was gentle, exploratory, and sensuous. If this had been a movie, they would have thrown off their clothes and made wild, passionate love in the woods. Jan was ambivalent because she felt loyalty to her boyfriend. Craig wanted a relationship with Jan, but worried it would turn into a triangle and a bad situation—he'd seen that happen too often with friends. They were holding hands when they walked out of the woods. Jan promised to call Craig if she chose to pursue the relationship. After soul-searching, talking with friends, and a sad and angry confrontation with the boyfriend, she called six days later.

Senior year is a time of major decisions and transitions, but what Jan and Craig remember were the delicious moments of their love affair. Jan used the birth control pill, so they began intercourse almost immediately. Their lovemaking consisted of much more than intercourse. There was lots of affection, especially kissing—which Craig particularly liked—and handholding—which was Jan's favorite medium to express affection. They watched videos or listened to tapes curled up in each others

arms. They caressed and stroked each other, clothed and un-
clothed. This kind of romantic love experience is special and not
to be missed. Craig enjoyed touching, nongenital as well as genital. When it culminated in intercourse, which was 90% of the
time, Craig was satisfied. Jan was open emotionally and sexually,
not a woman who played games. Craig believed she would be
loyal, and for the first time in his life was committed to being
sexually faithful. This was the most satisfying relationship Jan
ever experienced. She viewed Craig in a more idealized and romantic way than was true, as interested in emotional closeness
and affection as she was—the perfect man.

Craig was an engineering major and through a co-op program
was committed to working in another state. Jan had planned to
go to graduate school, but for the sake of the relationship chose
to postpone this and move with Craig. Although she is glad she
married Craig, Jan regretted the decision not to continue with
her career plans; she did not enter graduate school until thirteen
years later.

Living together is very different from dating. For Craig and
Jan, it was a difficult transition. There is the advantage of time
and privacy, but you have to deal with practical and mundane
matters, which makes time together less special. Sleeping in the
same bed each night is different. Romanticism and unpredictability is gone. This transition was harder for Jan than Craig. Jan's
parents were unhappy that she did not continue her education
and displeased about her living with a man. Jan's job was unsatisfying, and she did not like living in that town. Craig was
excited about his career, developing a mentor relationship with
the boss, and making friends with coworkers. Craig enjoyed the
regularity and stability of living together and the rhythm of intercourse four to five times a week. As often happens, special
moments and affection were taken for granted. Craig and Jan fell
into a sexual routine which was functional, but not special.

Touching and affection decreased, but intercourse remained
the same. This occurs with both nonmarital and marital couples.
It's not a conscious decision, just an easy trap to fall into. Although Jan was aware of dissatisfaction, it wasn't acute, so she
didn't voice her concerns. She felt better when Craig said, "Let's
get married before the end of the year, since we'll have to make
another move for my job."

Although people would claim there isn't much difference between living together and being married, that is not the reality for most couples, nor was it for Jan and Craig. Marriage is best viewed as a commitment to lead a life together and share plans, goals, values, and emotional and sexual intimacy. When Jan and Craig married it was with the hope and belief the marriage would be satisfying and secure. They were pleased to join their lives, emotionally, financially, and practically. Jan hoped with marriage there would be a return to affection and playfulness, but did not voice this. Unfortunately, affection and pleasure continued its downhill slide. It was not that Jan was dissatisfied with Craig, the marriage, or sex, but she missed touching, sensuality, and special moments.

Twelve years later Jan and Craig appeared at a therapist's office. The stated problem was concern over their nine-year-old son's school underachievement. The clinician did an evaluation of the entire family, not just the boy. She recommended tutoring in reading for the son and consultation concerning what the parents could do to increase academic motivation. They were pleased with those suggestions, but taken aback by the recommendation to seek marital therapy. The clinician felt Jan was depressed, and marital dissatisfaction was the cause. At first Jan was defensive, but on reflection admitted the assessment was correct. She was interested in discussing her concerns about life and the marriage with a therapist. Craig was considerably more reluctant, but was persuaded by the argument that relationship problems are more likely to be successfully resolved in couples therapy than in individual therapy and therapy would be effective in preventing a marital crisis. The child psychologist referred them to a marital therapist with a subspecialty in sex therapy.

The assessment format was to see Jan and Craig together, then each separately, and to have a couple feedback session to discuss issues and propose a course of treatment. Craig in his individual session stated few concerns. His primary complaint was that intercourse frequency had declined to once a week, typically on Saturday night, and almost always at his initiation. He rationalized that with their busy lives and schedules this was to be expected. Jan had more concerns and complaints. The primary one was the disappearance of affection, sensuality, and closeness. She enjoyed sex when they got around to it, but felt emotionally distant and not intimately connected. Jan felt the marriage was item ten on Craig's busy agenda, with the first seven items involving his job.

In the feedback session, the therapist said she was glad they'd come at this point because in another year the marriage would have been in crisis. She emphasized to both, but especially Craig, that this was the time to get the marriage back on track. She made a number of observations and suggestions, the most important involving couple time and nondemand touching. The easy, affectionate touching they'd experienced premaritally and early in the marriage had almost disappeared. There was little public affection other than routine kisses, and little cuddling or stroking except in bed on Saturday night, almost always foreplay for intercourse.

The therapist made it clear nondemand pleasuring was not a return to adolescent necking and petting games. It was a cooperative effort to revitalize affection and sensuality. While it is not appropriate to be sensual or sexual in front of children (these forms of sexual expression are private acts), it is a good sex education model for children to see their parents kissing, holding hands, hugging, and cuddling. Knowing that parents are loving and affectionate is reassuring for children. The therapist encouraged affectionate touching inside as well as outside the bedroom, to relearn that touch is critical for emotional bonding. Touch is not necessarily a signal or a demand for intercourse.

The therapist commented on Jan and Craig's almost total absence of sensuality. She suggested they take a bubble bath and/ or a relaxing, sensual shower together. This is something they had never done, not even in their early days. The novelty made it a special experience. Craig was out of touch with his sensual needs. He did enjoy washing Jan's back and Jan toweling him dry. For Jan these sensual experiences caused a reawakening of special feelings. Although the therapist made a point that sensuality was not meant to be a prelude to intercourse, it was Jan who initiated intercourse following the shower. Jan felt sensuous, desirous, and aroused. Intercourse was a natural continuation of those feelings. As they discussed that experience, there were several insights. Foremost was how important nondemand pleasuring was to Jan and how much she missed it. Craig acknowledged he'd enjoyed this and wanted pleasuring to be a part of their intimate relationship. Sensuality was an important bridge between affection and eroticism. A second discovery was how satisfying it was to engage in slow, nondemand touching and how important to connect emotionally and physically. Sensuality can have a strong effect on sexual desire, which was particularly striking to Jan. The therapist emphasized that although sensuality could and often does serve as an impetus for sex, it is not a demand. Sensuality works best in the context of a nondemand experience which is valued in and of itself. It serves as a bridge for intercourse when one partner is desirous and the other is open and receptive.

Jan and Craig learned that comfort with affection, sensuality, and intimacy is the basis of sexual desire. This is especially important for marriages of over two years duration.

NONDEMAND PLEASURING AS A BRIDGE TO INTERCOURSE

Nondemand pleasuring is the single most important component in sexual intimacy. It can and does serve a number of functions, one of which is a bridge for sexual desire. For many couples, it is their favorite way to initiate sex. For others, sensual experiences such as showers or baths, full-body massages, chest or back rubs, using lotion as an adjunct to touching, cuddling for ten minutes before going to sleep and on awakening, are bonding experiences. At times, this engenders desire, arousal, and a transition into intercourse. Sensuality serves as a bridge to intercourse when it is viewed as a couple process, not when one partner has a hidden agenda of wanting intercourse but is unwilling to ask. It is important that sex not be viewed as a teasing, withholding game. The decision to proceed to intercourse is a mutual one which evolves from the sensual interaction, from feeling responsive and turned on with a desire to extend this to intercourse.

For the typical couple, less than half of sensual experiences proceed to intercourse. Some couples engage in sensual experiences three to four times a week, others once a month. There is a positive relationship between openness to sensual experiences and frequency of intercourse. Sensuality fans the flames of desire and increases anticipation, connection, and arousal. Having a range of mutually acceptable ways to connect and express affection, sensuality, eroticism, and sexuality enhances marital intimacy.

An analogy couples find helpful is to a five-speed car. Gear 1 is clothes-on affectionate touching. Gear 2 is non-genital pleasuring, a sensual experience which can be semiclothed or nude. Gear 3 is playful touch, usually nude, which involves genital as well as non-genital pleasuring. Gear 4 is erotic stimulation (manual, oral, or rubbing) to high levels of arousal and orgasm (non-intercourse sex). Gear 5 involves intercourse and orgasm. Although many rides will involve all 5 gears, it isn't a requisite. Sometimes you just want a leisurely drive in the country. Each touching gear has value in itself. The touching experience needn't go to gear five to justify starting the car. Enjoy each affectionate, pleasuring, and erotic experience for itself.

Tina and Howard

It is nice to observe couples who have a comfortable sense of touch. You are most likely to see this among unmarried couples in their twenties—an old joke, that's not really funny, says you can tell married from unmarried people because married couples don't hold hands or touch in public.

Tina and Howard are in their late fifties and provide a powerful antidote to those perceptions. They enjoy being with each other, touching, and being touched. As Tina proudly says, "We come from touching families and our children touch in their marriages." What matters most are the small touches—stroking his cheek as Howard wakes up, a kiss that lingers a few seconds, Howard patting Tina on the bottom in the kitchen, a hug before leaving for work, teasing stroking of a breast or penis to carry a pleasing memory during the day, a gentle kiss when arriving home rather than a pro forma peck, a foot massage that creates nice sensations on Tina's tired feet, lying on the couch cuddling with intertwined legs, holding hands when going for a walk, taking a moment to sensuously caress the partner's face or arm, being easy and playful with touch, especially spontaneous touch.

Tina and Howard have their special scenario. Howard typically wakes early on Saturday morning. He enjoys feeding the animals, doing woodworking, and/or engaging in light exercise.

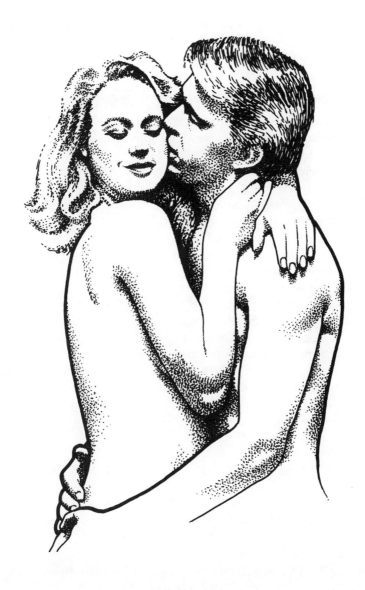

Nondemand pleasuring is the single most important component in sexual intimacy. Sensuality can be enjoyed for itself or can serve as a bridge to arousal and intercourse.

When Tina wakes she opens the door, which is a signal for Howard to put on the coffee. After a wake-up cup, they take a shower and towel each other dry. Tina checks that the children are still asleep, and Howard makes sure the phones are turned off. They lock the bedroom door to guard against unexpected interruptions.

Throughout the morning there have been light, teasing touches and jokes mixed with special looks. Tina enjoys Saturday morning sensual touching standing up rather than lying in bed. She especially enjoys kissing, caressing and playful genital touching in front of the bureau mirror. Visual feedback is erotic. One of the most sensuous elements is touching while semiclothed rather than nude—Tina puts on one of Howard's shirts and partially buttons it. Genital and nongenital pleasuring is intermixed. Howard will usually get an erection and Tina will feel turned on, but this is not a demand. Two of three Saturday mornings do include intercourse. Tina and Howard like the concept of intercourse as a "special pleasuring experience." Perhaps ten percent of the time they engage in manual, oral, or rubbing stimulation to orgasm as an alternative way to express eroticism. Other times are sensuous, relaxing, and comfortable and don't proceed to sex. Part of what makes this an inviting time for Tina is the unpredictability and variability. It's their special way to make the transition to the weekend, which, after Saturday morning, is filled with social, athletic, and family activities. This pattern developed when their children were school age and continues now when they have visiting grandchildren.

NONDEMAND PLEASURING DURING STRESSFUL TIMES

All couples go through stressful and taxing periods. External stressors may include a work deadline, illness or death of a parent, a child's academic problems, moving or home remodeling, a financial crisis, a period of depression or anxiety. There are times when one or both spouses simply do not feel sexual. Sexuality is not a biological need like food or drink. You can cease being sexual for months and nothing untoward will happen to your body. What can and does happen is a strain on the marital bond. One of the best ways to maintain an intimate connection during periods of nonsexuality, whether it extends over days, weeks, or months, is to continue affectionate touching and non-demand pleasuring.

Karen and Pete

Karen was being treated for back strain. During the treatment a medication was improperly administered and she was temporarily paralyzed. This was a very frightening experience. It took seven months before she was fully ambulatory. Karen was devoid of sexual feelings—she viewed her body with great concern, feeling it had betrayed her. However, needs for affection, especially her need to be held, were quite high. Pete was used to thinking of touching in sexual terms, so this forced experience of affectionate touching and massaging was new to him. Emotionally and physically Pete wanted to support Karen. Although they hope never to go through a period like that again, through it they became a closer couple. The experience opened Pete to the importance of touch as a means of communicating affection and support, and being there for Karen.

Sexual dysfunction or a nonsexual relationship strains a marital bond. Couples who maintain affectionate and sensual connection find this helps sustain motivation and emotional closeness. Couples who shut off all forms of physical communication are vulnerable to feelings of isolation and alienation. They are less motivated to deal with marital problems. In his clinical practice, Barry is encouraged when he sees couples who maintain a touching relationship. No matter how severe the sexual dysfunction, these couples have a better prognosis.

MALE-FEMALE DIFFERENCES IN NONDEMAND PLEASURING

It cannot be emphasized enough how the male-female premarital double standard interferes with communication between a husband and wife. In traditional male socialization, touch is sexual and goal-oriented. Traditionally, women have valued affectionate touch, but vetoed sexual activity. These rigid roles and definitions are antithetical to our concept of nondemand pleasuring being initiated by either partner. There is no place for hidden agendas, manipulation, or coercion. Nondemand pleasuring requires comfort and skill communicating your feelings and desires verbally and nonverbally. The spouse is free to communicate her feelings and wants. You trust the partner will respect your feelings. Men learn to value affectionate and sensual touch for itself, and women are comfortable with sexual initiation and the transition to arousal and intercourse. Conversely, a man needs to be comfortable saying no if he does not want to proceed to intercourse. He says no without feeling he's failed as a male. A woman can let go and be aware of the range of sensual and sexual feelings. She is not afraid he will push her, so she doesn't need to monitor his arousal. Ideally in a marital relationship both people can initiate, be open, say no, suggest alternatives, and enjoy affection, sensuality, eroticism, and intercourse. The nondemand pleasuring concept works best in the context of an emotionally intimate, equitable and secure relationship. Nondemand touching has a reciprocal function, both stimulating and reinforcing intimacy.

CLOSING THOUGHTS

Nondemand pleasuring builds and reinforces comfort with touch, sexual desire, receptivity to sexual stimulation, and emotional intimacy. It can serve as a bridge to arousal, intercourse, and orgasm. Nondemand pleasuring is a solid foundation for intimacy and sexuality. However, the traditional male objection is correct: nondemand pleasuring is not enough. Nondemand pleasuring is necessary, but not sufficient, for sexual satisfaction. The next chapter on eroticizing marriage will discuss erotic scenarios and techniques that are necessary but, without the base of nondemand pleasuring, difficult to integrate into marital sex.

4
EROTICIZING MARRIAGE

People seldom associate the term "erotic" with marital sex. Erotic is associated with new, intense relationships, whether premarital or extramarital. Erotica connotes the "fun, but dirty" sex found in X-rated movies, sex magazines, sex shops, and kinky sex. Can marital sex be erotic? Is this an unrealistic expectation? We are convinced—theoretically, empirically, and in terms of our own marriage—that marital sex can be exciting, erotic, and satisfying. We have been married thirty-one years and the quality of our sexual expression is higher than in the early years. Marital sex not only can be erotic, but eroticism is vital if you want to maintain pleasure, playfulness, and satisfaction.

Our prescription for marital sex is an emotionally intimate and secure bond with a solid foundation in nondemand pleasuring. Erotic scenarios and techniques are the additional ingredient that serves to make marital sex exciting and vital. Multiple stimulation, the most common erotic strategy, involves giving and/or receiving more than one type of sexual stimulation. In the "traditional" sexual scenario—although we don't believe many couples actually practiced this—the man stimulated the woman until she was sufficiently lubricated, then he initiated intercourse and thrusted until they had a simultaneous orgasm (viewed as "ideal sex"). Our guess is the "traditional" scenario worked for less than ten percent of couples.

COUPLE STRATEGIES AND TECHNIQUES

Each couple develops their own style of sexual expression. There is *not* "one right way" to eroticize marriage. We will examine guidelines used by couples who report a high degree of sexual satisfaction and suggest exercises developed in the context of sex therapy. This provides you with a smorgasbord of alternatives to discuss and experiment with. Choose sexual scenarios and techniques that enhance eroticism for you.

It is not technique alone, or even primarily, that eroticizes marital sex. Sexuality is enhanced by spontaneity, playfulness, and experimentation, but above all awareness of your feelings and openness to creative expression. Sexual creativity emanates from three sources: awareness of sexual feelings, fantasies, and desires; a dynamic view of the relationship, which includes touching and nonverbal communication; and an openness to experimenting with sexual scenarios and techniques. Creative sex involves awareness of feelings in the moment. Take the risk to convey these to your spouse and play them out. You don't need to give a Hollywood-level performance, but do need to share your body and feelings, express desires, and let go emotionally and sexually.

The death knell for sexuality is a routine, mechanical approach. The typical sexual scenario for married couples is sex at eleven or later at night. One person, usually the male, reaches over to kiss or caress and says, "Do you want to?" The sexual interaction follows a standard routine of five to ten minutes of foreplay, during which he gets her ready for intercourse; two to seven minutes of intercourse until the man and sometimes the woman reaches orgasm; a minute or two of hugging and talking, and then sleep. Is there something wrong with that scenario? No. However, it is not the stuff of a vital, satisfying sexuality. Why should sex be the last thing at night after you've finished all the important tasks of life, like paying bills, cleaning the house, putting children to sleep, and watching the late news? When sex has a low priority, it's hard for it to remain satisfying, much less erotic. A necessary component for erotic sex is setting aside time. You need to be alert and awake, value your time and privacy, and anticipate coming together for erotic sex.

Some people are offended by the concept of a "sexual date." They feel sex should be spontaneous. Spontaneity is fun, but in a couple's busy life, between children, jobs, household chores, community responsibilities, friends, and extended family, if you don't set aside couple time it won't happen. Couple time doesn't mean having sex each time, but does mean time to feel connected, without distractions. This allows you the opportunity to be sexual, but is not a sexual demand. Spontaneity works better in movies and novels than in a busy couple's life. It is easier to be spontaneous on vacations or weekends than at home during the busy week.

An interesting side note is that extramarital affairs thrive on excitement, anticipation, and eroticism. Yet an affair requires an enormous amount of planning and arrangement. You need to decide where to meet—often at a hotel or motel—and be assertive in asking for the "day rate." You block off time in the schedule, cover yourself at work, have someone pick up children, and plan what to tell your spouse if she asks. Not exactly a spontaneous coming together.

Spontaneity is fun and erotic, but its role is overemphasized. Spontaneous sexuality doesn't appear out of nowhere—there is a comfort with touching and intimacy which facilitates the transition to a passionate, erotic coming together.

A crucial concept is that sexual quality is more important than quantity. Couples—as in the Woody Allen classic movie *Annie Hall*—consistently battle over frequency of intercourse. These arguments are counterproductive and self-defeating. Sexual satisfaction is not measured by frequency or by the number of orgasms. The best measure of sexual satisfaction is a sense of giving and receiving pleasure and feeling bonded. This comes from quality, not quantity. Recalling special sexual experiences builds anticipation.

What makes for good sexual quality? An important component is developing and refining sexual scenarios. Each individual and couple has their favorite sexual scenario(s). Some people find the best time to be sexual is when they wake up. Others prefer sex after coffee and the morning paper. Others like a "nooner," before or after a nap, before dinner (sex as an appetizer) or after dinner (sex as dessert).

Part of the scenario is setting a mood. Couples set that mood by listening to music, going for a walk, talking about pleasant moments, having a glass of wine by candlelight, taking a bath together, having fifteen minutes of time alone and then coming together, or her meeting him at the door in a sexy outfit. Other couples prefer working in the garden, talking about feelings, or working out and then making the transition to being sexual. Many couples prefer to start the scenario outside the bedroom. They begin sensual touching and play in the living room and don't move into the bedroom until both are feeling turned on.

Once the scenario is initiated, couples choose different ways of playing it out. Remember, it's not a question of right or wrong, but of acting on your feelings, preferences, and desires. Some enjoy taking turns, others prefer mutual stimulation. Some people verbally express feelings and make requests. Others would rather let their fingers do the talking. Many couples prefer the scenario of moving from slow, tender, nongenital touching to light, playful, genital stimulation and then to focused, erotic stimulation, before proceeding to intercourse. Other couples begin intercourse as early as possible in the scenario. Most couples prefer multiple stimulation during the pleasuring period and intercourse itself. Others find it more erotic if the focus is on one form of stimulation at a time. For some, manual stimulation is most arousing, for others oral stimulation, and for others rubbing stimulation. Some couples prefer using one intercourse position, others change positions three times during intercourse. Creative sex involves awareness of your feelings and preferences. Develop and play out scenarios which are erotic for you. Quality depends on keeping open channels of sexual communication, whether by verbal requests, nonverbal hand-guiding, moving your body, or guiding the partner's mouth, hand, or body.

ORAL-GENITAL SEX

The major revolution in sexual technique has been experimentation with oral-genital sex. About 75 percent of married couples try oral sex and 40 percent regularly integrate oral sexuality into their lovemaking. This makes perfect sense—the mouth and genitals are the two parts of the body most capable of giving and receiving sexual pleasure. Couples who engage in oral sex report heightened sexual satisfaction, including enjoyment of intercourse.

Why does oral sex have a reputation as "kinky" or "dirty"?

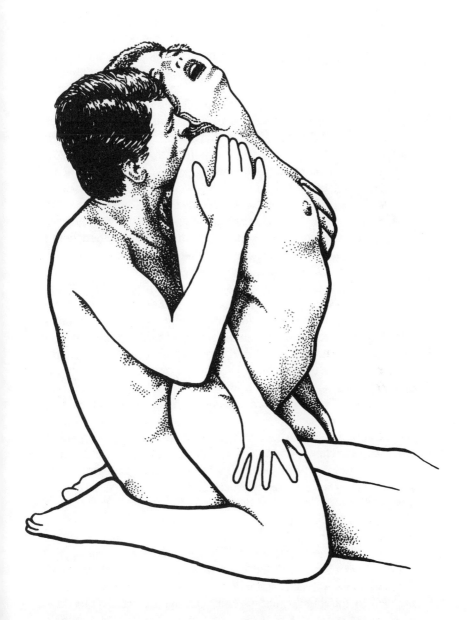

You can enjoy a range of sexual scenarios, positions and pleasuring techniques. Be open to trying different positions and types of pleasuring.

Much of the problem comes from our use, and misuse, of sexual language. The formal terms "cunnilingus" (his kissing, licking, or sucking her vulva) and "fellatio" (her kissing, licking, or sucking his penis) are cold, awkward Latin words. Slang phrases such as "blow job," "go down on," "suck off," "eat me," and "69" have hostile and/or derogatory connotations.

Oral sex has been viewed as "exciting, but dirty." Is it something you would do with an intimate partner? When married men go to prostitutes they pay more for fellatio than intercourse. Are their wives too inhibited to give oral sex, are men too embarrassed to ask, or do they believe only a prostitute could do it right? Males are too inhibited or embarrassed to request the spouse use harder or more rapid sucking. Men do not make specific requests such as a letting them thrust as they are being fellated or asking for additional stimulation like stroking the testicles or doing manual anal stimulation.

Some males believe only a man who is insecure about his penis would perform cunnilingus. The fear is a woman might become hooked on oral sex and forgo intercourse. Or the woman who has orgasms through cunnilingus can't have an orgasm during intercourse. What nonsense! You can develop comfort with cunnilingus and experiment with oral sex techniques which enhance eroticism and satisfaction.

In experimenting with oral sex, as with any sexual technique, a crucial guideline is to be open, but not allow coercion. Focus on pleasure, not performance. You don't need to prove anything to anybody. The best way to approach oral sex is gradually, intermixing oral with manual stimulation. We suggest bathing or showering together to avoid concern about cleanliness or genital smells. Couples who don't have time or want to bother with a shower can use a washcloth and deodorant soap to clean their genitals.

Begin with a giver-receiver format. The receiver can close his/her eyes, which reduces self-consciousness as well as helps you focus on pleasurable sensations. Begin oral stimulation with kissing before moving to licking and sucking. He can lightly kiss and run his tongue around the vulva, exploring the labia before focusing on the clitoral area. She might kiss and run her tongue along the shaft of the penis before kissing and sucking on the glans. The giver is free to experiment with a range of oral stim-

ulation techniques. If there is discomfort or pain, the recipient
needs to say that so the partner can change the stimulation. The
recipient enjoys the sensations and takes in pleasure.

Once you've established a basic comfort with giving and receiving oral stimulation, experiment with scenarios and positions
to build eroticism. Some people enjoy passively receiving, the
majority find it more arousing to move their body rhythmically
while being stimulated. Changing positions can increase erotic
feelings. Many women prefer the man to kneel beside her rather
than lie between her legs, so she feels connected and can touch
him. Many men prefer the position of man standing, woman
kneeling, because it gives him freedom to move and touch her
as she's stimulating him. Some couples enjoy mutual oral-genital
stimulation (the "69" position) as the ultimate in multiple stimulation, while others find it distracting to give and receive at the
same time. There is no right or wrong position or technique.
State your preferences, be aware of the partner's comfort, and
play until you develop a quality oral sex scenario(s).

A common fear among women is losing control or gagging
during fellatio. To prevent gagging we suggest two techniques.
Guide the penis to the side of your mouth, toward your cheek,
rather than putting it down the center. The second is to keep
your hand on the penis so insertion is not too deep or fast. Holding his penis gives you a sense of control as well as providing
additional stimulation.

Is oral sex a pleasuring technique or do you want to proceed
to orgasm? Being orgasmic during cunnilingus facilitates arousal
during intercourse. The most common method of achieving multiorgasmic response is cunnilingus. Many women find it easier
to be orgasmic with cunnilingus than intercourse. Some find if
they're orgasmic with cunnilingus it's easier to be orgasmic during intercourse.

Fellatio to orgasm is a sensitive issue. If the male ejaculates
during fellatio he will not be able to engage in intercourse. An
emotionally charged issue is whether the man will ejaculate in
the woman's mouth. For some couples this is comfortable and
the woman swallows the semen (semen is hygienically safe and
even low caloric). Some women do fellatio to orgasm, but prefer
to spit out the semen rather than swallow it. Other women find
the sensation of semen gushing into their mouth unpleasant. In-

stead, the man withdraws and ejaculates on the sheet, on her, or himself. Other couples prefer to use fellatio only as a pleasuring technique and proceed to intercourse.

Oral sex enhances the quality of marital sex and facilitates creative, erotic sexuality. The couple is aware of feelings and desires, communicates these verbally and nonverbally, develops oral sex scenarios that are comfortable and erotic, and creatively integrates oral sex into their lovemaking.

Sandi and Jack

Couples who find sex easy from the beginning need to be aware of the potential trap of taking it for granted and allowing the sexual relationship to stagnate. Sandi met Jack when she was twenty-three and he twenty-four. Prior dating and sexual experiences followed the typical roller-coaster pattern of excitement and anticipation at the beginning, highs and lows throughout, and pain and hurt at the breakup.

When Sandi and Jack met at a wedding, each felt ready for a serious relationship. Although they still disagree about who pursued whom, the first two months were romantic and erotic. Romantic love is a special experience not to be missed, although it is not a good basis for marital choice. This is a passionate, fun time, full of erotic sex and idealization of the person and relationship. Sandi and Jack did special things lovers do—called at three in the morning, made love in the woods on a camping trip, stayed up all night sharing hopes and dreams, had sex three times a day, and swore they'd never hurt or disappoint the other. Romantic love is an exhilarating experience, but it's based on a fantasy assumption about the partner, love, and sex. Romantic love seldom lasts even for a year. Sandi looks back on those months more wistfully than Jack, although he too has fond memories.

After the romantic love phase evolved into mature, stable intimacy, sexuality remained easy and high quality. Both experienced sexual desire, although Jack's was more readily elicited. Both were easily aroused, receptive and responsive to stimulation, and one's arousal turned on the other. Orgasm was readily achieved, although on occasion Jack would ejaculate earlier than desired. In those cases, he would manually stimulate Sandi to orgasm. After sex they felt warm and bonded. Their marriage day was a true celebration with family and friends. Getting pregnant was not a problem; they had a girl and boy, and then Jack had a vasectomy. Life sailed along and they were viewed as a "golden couple."

One of the realities of life is, hard times come to all couples. You cannot avoid difficulties, and it's no use pretending they're not happening. Ideally, you would accept the reality, cope with the situation, and solve the problem with the spouse.

In an eight-month period Sandi's mother died, their son broke his arm, Jack's business was in a trough and he had to take a significant pay cut, and Sandi had a short affair with a doctor she'd met at the hospital emergency room. The affair came to light when Jack discovered her diaphragm and confronted her, since he'd had a vasectomy. The marital bond, especially trust, was damaged. An extramarital affair plunges the marriage into crisis. The wife having an affair is a reversal of the male-female double standard. The husband reacts as if it's an attack on his masculinity and sexual adequacy.

Jack was hurt and angry. Coming on top of career and financial setbacks, he felt vulnerable and insecure. Sandi also felt vulnerable, the affair had been impulsive. She regretted it and was apologetic. She was distressed by Jack's feelings of betrayal and the damage to their marital bond. The better the marriage, the more negative is the impact of an affair.

Sandi and Jack found the next three months the hardest of their marriage. In addition to dealing with other issues, they had to work through feelings of betrayal, anger, and depression; and rebuild the trust bond. Sex during those three months was particularly difficult. Like many married couples, Sandi and Jack had treated their sexual relationship with benign neglect. Sex is like a garden, it needs consistent attention and care. Sex was not dysfunctional, but had settled into a routine: less frequent, late at night, with less feeling and few special experiences. Sex following the revelation of the affair was sometimes angry, as if Jack was trying to get back at Sandi, with hard, rapid thrusting as his weapon. Other times there was a tentativeness that made them feel as if they were "walking on eggshells." Comfortable, easy sex was gone.

Although a crisis hastens the demise of unselfconscious sexual expression, the truth is, this eventually disappears from even the best marriage. Sandi and Jack were abruptly confronted with a transition all couples need to face—how to integrate creative, vital sex into an ongoing marriage. Rather than returning to the "good old days," they were better advised to focus on developing a couple sexual style that was high quality and would nurture their marital bond.

For Sandi and Jack, as with other couples in crisis, seeking marital therapy was the best thing to do. Therapy helped them deal with the affair, and more importantly, mobilized them to revitalize their bond. The therapist's first suggestion was to put a temporary prohibition on intercourse and reintroduce nongenital pleasuring. Sandi found that Jack's touching in a warm, tender, nondemanding manner renewed her attraction and desire to be with him. At first, Jack had difficulty being open to Sandi's touch. As he did, resentment dissipated. Nondemand touching and increased intimacy were the foundation for their revitalized sexual bond.

Genital pleasuring was reintroduced a week before the therapist lifted the ban on intercourse. This allowed Sandi and Jack to experiment with erotic stimulation to orgasm, something they had not done since their premarital years. Nondemand pleasuring builds comfort and sensuality. Playful and creative genital pleasuring adds eroticism and adventure. The genuine enjoyment of erotic scenarios and techniques made for a very sexual week. Even without intercourse, or maybe because there was a ban on intercourse, their sexual expression was more creative and erotic than it had been for years. Jack discovered a pleasuring position in which they both knelt on the bed, facing each other. This allowed him to engage in oral breast stimulation combined with manual clitoral stimulation while she manually stimulated him. For the first time in their marriage, Sandi was multiorgasmic. Although Jack was embarrassed about ejaculating in her hand, the sensations of direct stimulation to orgasm were exciting and gratifying.

When the therapist lifted the ban on intercourse she suggested Sandi and Jack think of intercourse as a special pleasuring technique. Eroticizing marriage means incorporating multiple stimulation throughout lovemaking, before and during intercourse. She warned them not to revert to the standard "foreplay" routine, but to continue with creative pleasuring scenarios, positions, and techniques. Intercourse was a natural extension of the pleasuring process.

The second focus was continuing multiple stimulation during intercourse. Sandi particularly desired manual clitoral stimulation in combination with intercourse. She also enjoyed kissing during coital thrusting and having her breasts caressed. Jack found it arousing to look at Sandi as she became aroused. Also, Jack enjoyed utilizing sexual fantasies. Marital sex benefits from erotic stimulation during intercourse.

TAKING RISKS WITH THE SPOUSE

Sexual desires, fantasies, and feelings are among the most private and sensitive aspects of human existence. Sharing these in the context of an intimate marriage is special. People fear rejection, worrying their requests will be perceived as "kinky" or perverse. We encourage couples to openly share sexual feelings and requests. A key in intimacy is trusting the partner and making clear, direct sexual requests—but she needs to hear it as a request, not a demand. This gives the spouse freedom to say, "Let's try it," offer an alternative erotic technique, or say, "No, I'm not comfortable with this." For example, a woman had read about being stimulated by a feather and was interested in trying this, but the husband disliked feathers. He suggested instead rubbing a string of pearls over her body. A man wanted his hands and feet tied with heavy rope, but the spouse suggested instead knots made with yarn. Don't do something which feels coercive or causes pain. Within those guidelines there are a wide variety of scenarios, positions, and techniques to explore. Sexual risks pay dividends in high-quality, erotic marital sex.

Jill and Ron

This was a couple who tried to "keep up with the Joneses," whether buying video equipment, seeing the most avant-garde play, reading trendy novels, or trying the newest gourmet cuisine. Each year, as soon as they read or heard about a new sexual scenario, they would try it. First it was anal intercourse, then use

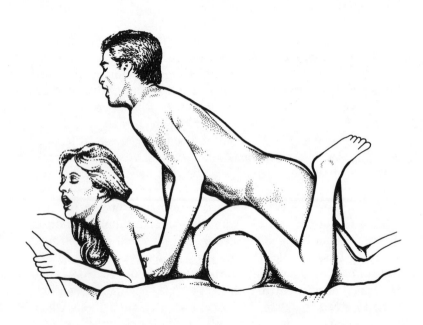

You can use pillows or cushions to increase comfort and sensations during rear-entry intercourse. Don't be afraid to experiment with your intimate partner.

of fruit-flavored creams with oral sex, then X-rated videos to use during lovemaking, followed by X-rated motels with Jacuzzis, vibrating beds, and ceiling mirrors. Last year it was playing out sexual fantasies with all the accouterments, including clothing and music. Still, Jill and Ron felt their sex life was stale, and were on the lookout for the next esoteric sexual scenario.

When they discussed this with a friend who was a marital therapist, she pointed out that these techniques made their sex life exciting for only a short time. Jill and Ron substituted external stimulation for an exploration of internal feelings and what they really wanted from each other. The next day Jill suggested taking a walk and talking. Ron, on the defensive, said their friend was an old-fashioned, uptight mental-health type. Jill agreed, but the more she thought about it the more she realized she wasn't doing what she wanted. They would try something for a while, then drop it. Why was that? As Ron thought about it, he realized what he liked best was having his testicles stroked while Jill orally stimulated him. Yet she hadn't done that in over a year and he hadn't asked her to. Jill said the scenario she liked best was pretty basic: lying on her back with Ron kneeling over her rubbing his penis against her breast while manually stimulating her clitoris. She felt embarrassed at desiring something so "vanilla," so didn't request it. Jill and Ron needed to accept that the essence of creative, erotic sexuality is being aware of feelings and preferences, not learning some exotic or sophisticated technique. Jill said it best: "We were so focused on trying to prove we were sexually liberated that we stopped communicating our intimate sexual needs."

CLOSING THOUGHTS

The key to eroticizing marriage is communicating sexual feelings and requests and developing your couple sexual style. We encourage an attitude of experimentation with sexual scenarios, positions, and techniques, especially multiple stimulation during intercourse. Creative, high-quality sexuality is much more than technique. Be aware of your feelings and erotic preferences and communicate these. The combination of emotional intimacy, pleasuring, and erotic stimulation is the best way to maintain vital, satisfying marital sex.

5

EQUITY BETWEEN THE SEXES

Among single people the "Dating Game" is more like the "War between the Sexes." A tragedy for American couples is that self-defeating attitudes, behavior, and emotional reactions learned premaritally sabotage the marriage.

What is needed is a new model of female-male relationships which facilitates respect, trust, and intimacy. The traditional double standard held that men and women were different, especially sexually, and needed to assume separate and rigid roles in marriage. A best-selling pop psychology book talks about men and women being from different planets. What nonsense!

We are unequivocally opposed to the double standard. It fosters a climate of disrespect, miscommunication, and distrust. Its only advantage is the rules about male-female roles are simple and clear, although wrong and harmful. The radical feminist standard of absolute equality between women and men, with everything split fifty-fifty, sets unrealistic expectations and results in constant power struggles. The male is viewed as the "bad guy." Traditional men call those who cave in to feminist demands "wimps." The radical feminist approach downplays trust and intimacy and overemphasizes personal independence and taking power. This makes for better political polemics than a model for an intimate and secure marriage. The equity model conceptualizes female-male relationships in a manner that enhances psychological and sexual well-being for men and women and facilitates a respectful, trusting, and intimate marriage.

A MODEL OF EQUITY BETWEEN WOMEN AND MEN

The foundation is: each spouse brings to the relationship the self-concept of deserving respect, being trustworthy, autonomous, competent, and sexual. You cannot expect the partner to give this to you. It's your responsibility to develop positive self-esteem, including sexual self-esteem. Healthy marriages are based on a positive influence model, which brings out the best in you as a person.

This model does not promote equality in every aspect of life, which is idealistic and doomed to failure. A solid, realistic base is a sense of equity in the marriage. One spouse has prime responsibility and skill in specific areas while the other has prime responsibility and skill in other areas. The crucial element is that the couple relate as respectful human beings who value each other's competence and share power in an equitable manner. When the couple relate as respectful, trusting, and caring people, they offer an excellent model from which children can learn about female-male roles and marriage. An added bonus is that people who treat each other well outside the bedroom will treat each other well inside the bedroom.

Respect is the cornerstone of the equity model. You have to respect yourself and the way you are in the marriage as well as respecting the spouse. When respect erodes, the marital bond is in danger. Respect is based on genuine knowledge of yourself and the spouse; you are accepted for your weaknesses and vulnerabilities as well as your strengths and competencies.

The second dimension involves trust. Instead of a war between the sexes with each jealously guarding his/her turf, in a trusting relationship you have confidence the spouse would not do something to purposely undercut or hurt you. You believe he has your best interests at heart, he's your friend and supporter. This does not mean returning to the traditional traps of a woman naively accepting everything a man does and him putting her on a pedestal. Discuss and reach an explicit agreement about what you mean by the trust bond and how important trust is in the marriage. Too many wives have felt victimized by husbands they naively believed and who took advantage of them. Too many husbands have felt devastated and abandoned by wives who they believed would love and stand by them no matter what.

This process begins before marriage. Choose a spouse who is

deserving of trust. Have a clear understanding about the importance of trust in the marital bond. Trust is not something you can or should take for granted, it needs to be developed, and its importance reinforced. For trust to be genuine, it must be reciprocal.

Even with a strong trust bond, at times there will be problems, disappointments, and anger. Dealing with hard issues and disagreements is a natural part of sharing your lives. That is the reality of the complex process of marriage. In dealing with mundane as well as major issues, each person needs to communicate clearly, discuss feelings and perceptions, suggest alternatives, and solve problems so agreements are reached that both can live with. In dealing with emotionally difficult issues, it is crucial that you trust the spouse's intentions. Refrain from doing something that intentionally hurts the partner or your marital bond.

Discussions can break down into power struggles where you care more about the fight than preserving the fabric of the relationship. When power struggles degenerate, they become "pissing contests." The issue is no longer important, what's important is not losing. Power struggles are destructive to the trust bond.

Couples can deal with difficult issues and reach agreements that reinforce rather than damage the trust bond. State your feelings, perceptions, and requests in a clear and assertive manner without putting down or threatening the spouse. Negotiating and problem solving does not break trust as long as you act in your best interest and don't try to intimidate or coerce the spouse. Do not negotiate so you win the battle but lose the war for the relationship. You want to reach an equitable agreement. Ideally, you would feel good about the process and outcome. Minimally, you can live with the agreement.

Trust means more than not having an extramarital affair. Sexual fidelity is not the only, or even the most important, element in marital trust. Extramarital affairs are a highly emotional and value-laden topic, which we discuss in detail in Chapter 17. We suggest developing a clear agreement regarding extramarital affairs.

The third important component is intimacy. Traditional, as well as modern, mythology holds that men and women are very different creatures when it comes to emotional and sexual expression. Women are purported to be more sensitive, empathic, able to express sadness, and dependent on being in a loving relationship in order to feel sexual. Men are purported to value control and rationality, able to express only anger, and value sexuality more highly than anything else in marriage. Women are said to value love and allow sex, and men to value sex and allow marriage in order to obtain sex. What rubbish!

The equity model promotes each spouse being comfortable in both emotional and sexual domains. Each person is capable of self-disclosure, able to express a range of feelings, share perceptions, solve problems, reach agreements, and be emotionally open and vulnerable. Emotional expression can be deep and stable as well as loving and intense. Marriage involves sharing your lives, including emotional and sexual intimacy.

Sexuality is a crucial element in intimacy. Sexuality includes sharing attraction, thoughts, feelings, beliefs, touching, and values, as well as intercourse and orgasm. Sexual intimacy is a vital, integral component of marriage. Sex can reinforce and deepen intimacy, is a shared pleasure, and serves as a tension reducer or safety valve. But, contrary to the media myth, it is not the most important element in a marriage. When sex goes well, it's 15 to 20 percent of the marriage, with its most important function being to energize the marital bond and make it special. It is only when sex is dysfunctional, nonexistent or part of a power struggle, that it plays an inordinately powerful role (50 to 75 percent), robbing the relationship of intimacy and draining loving feelings.

Sexuality works best where there is an equitable marriage. Each partner feels comfortable initiating (this is particularly hard for women) and each feels free to say no (this is particularly hard for men). Sex is more than genitals, intercourse, and the 3 to 10 seconds of orgasm. Sexuality involves acceptance of yourself as a sexual person, comfort with nondemand touching inside and outside the bedroom, enjoyment of sensuality, responsivity to genital stimulation and feeling turned on, openness to erotic scenarios and techniques, the ability to let go and be orgasmic, and afterplay and feeling bonded. Sex serves as an important expression of intimacy. It has been said that "a marriage can tolerate bad sex, but it's hard to survive no sex." The partners view each other as sexual people with sexuality integrated into a respectful, trusting, intimate marriage.

EQUITY GUIDELINES

The most intimate and stable relationship between a woman and a man is marriage. Although elements of the equity model are relevant to a range of relationships, including work colleagues, friendships, parenting and other social and family relationships, it is most crucial in marriage. These are guidelines for equity between the sexes:

1. Relationships between women and men are based on respectful attitudes that promote, and even demand, equity.
2. Develop open and flexible attitudes toward female-male roles.
3. Be accepting and secure about your femininity or masculinity. You do not need the approval of others, nor are you intimidated by rigid sex roles.
4. Be aware that intellectually, behaviorally, emotionally, and sexually there are more similarities than differences between women and men.
5. Encourage personal and/or professional friendships with the opposite sex, resist the pressure to sexualize these relationships.
6. Be comfortable and confident in your femininity or masculinity so activities and interests which have traditionally been labeled as belonging to the opposite sex can be integrated into your life.
7. An intimate sexual relationship is more satisfying if both the woman and man can initiate, say no, request, and value sexual pleasure.
8. Conception, contraception, and children are as much the responsibility of the man as the woman.
9. A respectful, equitable, trusting and intimate marriage is the most satisfying.
10. A communicative, sharing, and giving relationship promotes emotional and sexual satisfaction.

Couples who live out these guidelines, sharing responsibility to implement them, will avoid the war between the sexes and enjoy a satisfying and stable marriage.

DIFFERENCES BETWEEN WOMEN AND MEN

Much of the discussion and writing concerning female-male roles has been ideological, moralistic, and highly emotional. It generates much heat, but little light. Let us approach this complex subject from an objective, scientific viewpoint. There has been a great deal of scientific research during the past twenty-five years about female-male similarities and differences along a number of dimensions—physical strength, intellectual functioning, behavioral characteristics, health, sexual response, emotional reactivity, and interpersonal traits. The objective evidence is overwhelming: there are many more similarities than differences between women and men in all dimensions, including sexual response. The same phases of desire, arousal, orgasm, and emotional satisfaction are experienced by both women and men. The same psychological process of positive anticipation, the same physiological process of vasocongestion (accumulation of blood) and myotonia (muscle tension), the same rhythmic contractions of orgasm, and the same resolution period occurs for women and men. Of course there are differences, but the similarities—physically, psychologically, and emotionally—vastly outnumber them.

The main sexual differences involve latency of response and variability of orgasm. Women require a longer period of time and more direct genital stimulation for arousal than men, although these differences decrease with age and experience. Female orgasmic response is more flexible and variable. The male has a single orgasm during intercourse, which is accompanied by ejaculation. The woman might be nonorgasmic, singly orgasmic, or multiorgasmic. This can occur in the pleasuring/foreplay period, during intercourse, or in the afterplay phase. This does not mean female sexual response is better or worse than male, but it is more complex and variable. The important similarity is both women and men are sexual people with the ability to give and receive pleasure, be orgasmic, and value sexuality.

Marlene and Paul

Few couples have benefited from growing up in families where there was an equitable model between mother and father.

Marlene and Paul were in the majority who hoped to develop a marital bond which was very different from that of their parents.

Marlene was ten when her parents separated. She observed the three-year agony of trying to reconcile, angrily parting, and trying again. Father left for the final time when she was thirteen, after a violent confrontation in which Mother called the police— she had done so previously, but this time followed through with legal charges. Marlene had minimal contact with her father until she was twenty-two. He had remarried and his life was more stable, although he would still lose his temper and lash out at his new wife and child. Marlene saw her father as financially successful, but as a man who was dependent on a woman to keep his life under control. She resented his temper and was frightened by it. Marlene feared men would use physical intimidation and anger to get their way. She was empathic with her mother, although as an adolescent used Mother's emotional weakness as leverage to get her way. In retrospect, Marlene was not proud of her adolescent behavior.

Like other children of divorce, Marlene had a strong need to marry and develop a more stable life than she experienced growing up. Yet negative motivation seldom, if ever, promotes positive behavior. Marlene's marriage at twenty-one was a badly thought-out choice. One of the reasons children of divorce have higher divorce rates is that they marry young and idealize their partner as the perfect romantic love object. Marriage, however, is a rational and emotional commitment to sharing your life, and romantic love subverts a mature, realistic marital choice.

Eight months into the marriage, Marlene was badly disillusioned and scared. She admired Mother for seeking therapy after the divorce; individual and group therapy made her a stronger person. Marlene entered individual psychotherapy when her husband adamantly refused to seek marital therapy. The therapist was respectful and empathic with Marlene, but confrontative about her taking responsibility for decisions, evaluating her reasons for marrying, and assessing the viability of her marriage. The therapist suggested Marlene talk to Mother and Father to obtain information and consultation, but not blame them for the state of her life or have them make decisions for her. Each parent was supportive and neither pressed her to stay in this marriage.

Being in individual therapy to improve a marriage can be help-ful to the individual, but usually increases marital dissatisfaction. Marlene's husband made fun of therapy and blamed all marital problems on her "immaturity" and "selfishness." Marlene was aware enough to refuse the blame, and resentful because he wouldn't consider the problems as a couple issue. After con-sulting with friends, family, and the therapist, Marlene decided that rather than allow the relationship to deteriorate further, in-creasing the pain and letting life get more out of control, she had to confront the reality that this was a fatally flawed marriage. Although the outcome was sad and the transition to being single again difficult, Marlene didn't regret her decision. She was glad she lived at a time when women were responsible for themselves and didn't have to cling to a destructive marriage. Marlene did not need a man in her life in order to feel like a complete person.

A year and a half after the divorce she met Paul. In choosing to remarry, she had learned from the past and this time was ready to make a marital commitment for the right reasons. Paul too had a poor parental model, although his parents remained mar-ried. He had read about abusive husbands in magazine articles and seen them depicted on television and in movies, but had not heard or read about abusive wives and mothers. Yet this was the reality of his family. Although both parents denied it, alcoholism and drug abuse were central problems. Paul's father functioned at work, but used alcohol to shut off his feelings and avoid deal-ing with the destructive marital and family dynamics. Paul saw his father as a nice person, but too weak to confront difficult, if not impossible, issues. Paul was extremely frightened of his mother. Every two weeks she would fly into a rage (caused in part by mixing alcohol and drugs), often accompanied by vio-lence toward the husband or children. This could result in any-thing from a broken chair to a broken arm. Neighbors called the police, who left after things calmed down. Paul's psychological scars from this violence were deeper and more lasting than the scar he bore on his arm. He was determined to never become caught in an abusive relationship with a woman.

As a young adult, Paul attended meetings of and read material about Adult Children of Alcoholics. This increased his awareness and decreased the stigma, but Paul was not impressed with the people in the group, he felt they wallowed in their role as victim. He was wary of commitments, although he enjoyed dating, sexuality, and "light" relationships.

Marlene and Paul met through mutual friends who encouraged them to volunteer for a Special Olympics project. Marlene was attracted to the open and engaging manner Paul displayed with retarded children. Paul found Marlene very attractive. She seemed competent and self-possessed even when everything around her was chaotic. After the day's activities, a group of volunteers went to a bar to socialize, and Marlene and Paul joined them. Paul noted that she limited herself to two drinks, as did he. He was impressed by how sociable and down to earth she was. Marlene liked Paul, but was not as taken with him as he was with her.

In a relationship, someone has to take the risk and be the pursuer. In our culture it is usually the man. Paul asked for Marlene's phone number and called the next day. Marlene had a preference for informal first dates during daylight hours, so she suggested they meet for lunch. Although Paul had suggested a movie, he agreed to lunch. First dates are some of the best and worst parts of being single. They can be disappointing and tiresome. Going through the routine of exchanging information about where you live, your work, where you're from, etc., can be tedious. On the positive side, there's a sense of anticipation, excitement, adventure, and hope this could turn into something special.

Marlene and Paul approached their relationship cautiously. They had fun getting to know each other. They enjoyed touching and affection, but neither was in a rush to sexualize the relationship. Neither trusted romantic love feelings or intense emotional expression. At the very least, Marlene wanted to be sure Paul would be a good and trustworthy friend. Paul was wary of Marlene's turning into an explosive, unpredictable person.

When their children are old enough to ask about their parents' courtship, the story Marlene and Paul will share begins with a Friday night movie that was so bad they left in the middle. It was a pleasant fall night, so they took a walk along the river. They discussed mental retardation caused by fetal alcohol syndrome. Before he knew it, Paul was talking about this in a very personal manner, relating it to his family experience. His self-disclosure was not an emotional outburst; he asked whether Marlene was interested in hearing the story. They walked and talked for over two hours. This established a pattern that was to last throughout their marriage. Paul found it easier to discuss emotional issues while engaged in an activity like walking, raking leaves or working on a household project. Marlene was an empathic listener, attending to his story and emotions rather than feeling sorry for him or rushing in to make him feel better. She disclosed one thing about herself that really struck Paul—she believed in marriage and wanted children, but wanted a husband who was as complete a person as she was. Paul appreciated her strength and was relieved that she did not exhibit the desperateness he saw in so many divorced women. The second part of the walk was quieter, with kissing and touching. They wanted to make love, which Marlene acknowledged. However, she did not want to add a sexual dimension to this already full day. Marlene invited him to spend the night Saturday, after they'd had time to think things out and only if Paul were open to a serious relationship.

This would not sell as a romantic novel, but does make a healthy start for an intimate relationship. Paul brought a change of clothes as well as condoms. Marlene preferred to use a diaphragm, but not until they had a frank conversation about any risk of sexually transmitted disease, including HIV. She suggested they have sex before dinner. She wasn't looking for a great sexual performance, but an exploration and an introduction.

Once the sense of newness and illicitness wears off, it takes couples at least six months to develop a sexual style that is satisfying for both partners. Marlene and Paul were lucky in that they brought to the relationship positive sexual attitudes, awareness and comfort, and receptivity and responsivity to touch. Sexuality was easy for them, but unlike romantic love couples, they did not take it for granted.

After partners get married, they have a tendency to allow the sexual relationship to rest on its laurels. Marlene and Paul wanted to enhance sexuality so it would energize their marital bond as well as provide special moments and memories. Both felt free to initiate, and either could say no and offer an alternative. They engaged in nondemand touching both inside and outside the bedroom. Marlene and Paul enjoyed sensual activities such as showering together and using a lotion to enhance body massages. They were open to sexual scenarios in which one person was the giver as well as mutual, interactive scenarios. They enjoyed multiple stimulation, both before and during intercourse. Not all touching led to intercourse. They used a variety of intercourse positions with a range of scenarios from "quickies" to romantic, prolonged lovemaking. They accepted variability in sexual expression—sometimes sex was satisfying for both, sometimes one enjoyed it more than the other. When sex was mediocre or poor they laughed it off rather than blaming the other or worrying. They also enjoyed a range of afterplay experiences. Equity between the woman and man occurs both inside and outside the bedroom.

Their decision to marry did not follow the traditional romantic script. Marlene and Paul talked about strengths as well as potential problems areas. She needed assurance that Paul was committed to making the marriage successful, and he needed assurance that Marlene's interest was genuine and would not change with marriage. They would not tolerate the unsatisfying patterns of their parents' marriages—they would not stay married if the relationship became destructive. This solution was not used as a way out, but as positive motivation to maintain a viable marital bond. Marriage and sexuality is a process, not a product—it requires continual time, energy, commitment, and openness to personal and couple growth.

The decision to marry is based on both emotional and rational factors. In addition to intimacy and sexual attraction, you commit to building a satisfying life together. Marlene and Paul talked about a five-year plan for their lives and marriage: where they would live, how they would handle career and money issues, waiting at least two years before having a child, both would be actively involved in parenting, each had freedom to pursue individual interests and friends but not have sexual affairs or do anything that was detrimental to the marriage. They discussed hard issues such as the psychological "traps" from their parents' marriages, Marlene's divorce, Paul's fear of commitment, contact with extended family, how to deal with conflict and reach agreements, and the difficulties inherent in balancing individual interests, two careers, their marital bond, and parenting. Love is *not* enough for a successful marriage. Both partners need to be aware and committed to deal with issues, talk out problems before they lead to emotional alienation or a crisis. There are no perfect people or perfect marriages. Marlene and Paul had a strong commitment to make their marriage equitable, satisfying, and stable.

Marlene and Paul have been married eighteen years. Their daughter Teresa is fifteen and their son Mike twelve. They emphasize equity in their marriage. Sometimes it has worked "like in the book." The best example is that Paul's career has progressed better than either would have predicted. He was in a position to take more risks since Marlene's job as a bank operations officer provided a steady source of income. Paul has an advanced degree in biomedical engineering and developed instrument patents which he sold to a hospital supply company. He and Marlene respect each other's professional competence, and approach financial matters as a team.

The area in which equity guidelines worked least well involved household chores. Paul did not keep his agreements about cooking and housecleaning. In truth, he was a terrible cook. On his nights to cook they invariably had carry-out food or salads from the grocery store. Marlene was not happy about this, but realized it was unlikely to change. The guidelines worked well around parenting. Paul was a more involved and responsible parent than he imagined he could be. He felt equally comfortable nurturing as providing discipline. This freed Marlene to expand her role to roughhousing and teaching the children money management. Marlene enjoyed parenting and saw Paul as a fully participating father. Their parental bond reinforced their marital bond. They found parenting adolescents difficult, but viewed this as a challenge.

Not all couples can develop and implement equity guidelines as successfully as Marlene and Paul, yet the equity model is relevant for most marriages.

MIDDLE YEARS MARRIAGES

As a couple approaches their fortieth birthdays, new issues arise. They have been married between ten to fifteen years. If they are going to make major changes in their lives or marriages, this is the time to do so. Some couples find this period particularly rocky, and consider separation or divorce. Often the issue is the woman growing independent and assertive, becoming more involved in her career or community. The man has risen to a certain level in his career and is more interested in devoting time and energy to his wife and family. Couples find that their personal interests and goals are no longer complementary. This can lead to misunderstanding, conflict, and emotional distance, as well as feeling unappreciated and unloved.

Ann and Ken

This couple was feeling good about their growth and development until Ken was forty-three and Ann forty-one. Ten years ago, after the birth of their second child, they experienced stress and sought marital therapy. They remained in therapy for over a year, exploring feelings, learning communication skills, identifying destructive patterns, and discussing personal growth within the marriage. In the past year, they joined a marital enrichment program sponsored by their church. Ken and Ann were considered by many to be an ideal couple.

When the children entered elementary school, Ann returned to school and completed a Masters degree. She had been working full-time for three years, and been promoted twice. She found herself bringing home a great deal of work, and traveling on a regular basis. Ken had reached a middle management position in which he felt stable and secure, although not satisfied. Over the past five years, he had consciously moderated his work load and drastically reduced out-of-town travel. He became active around the home and coached his son's baseball team. Clearly they were at different places in their interests: Ann putting a lot of herself into her career, Ken wanting to emphasize home and family. Ken's changes were in response to Ann's request that he not be so work- and performance-oriented. He resented her doing what he had done ten years before. She was less available to share companionship, as a parent and an energetic sex partner. He felt cheated and resentful, and reacted by distancing himself. Ann was feeling a combination of exhilaration and guilt. She enjoyed her career, feelings of competence, and friendships with colleagues. Yet she worried that the children and Ken were feeling slighted and resented that becoming her own person meant she had to deal with feelings of guilt and pressure from husband and family.

For six months their marriage endured a painful period dominated by resentment. They were no longer the ideal couple, but continued to participate in couple activities, which helped them through this difficult transition. Especially helpful was a weekly sex life and the enjoyment of family activities. The marriage survived personal changes they underwent while maintaining their intimate bond.

There were no simple solutions for Ken and Ann. They needed to state desires, plans, and fears, listen without being defensive, and negotiate agreements. Ann wanted to be free of guilt feelings. Ken agreed to cease critical comments as long as Ann was honest with him about her plans and time constraints. Ann realized that when she made promises she couldn't keep, Ken got angry and she felt guilty. Ken came to accept that his involvement with the children and home were in his best interest, he was not doing them to please Ann. His desire for her to return to their previous lifestyle was unrealistic and inappropriate. Each person changes and every marriage changes. You have to live your lives as they are now; you can't turn the clock back.

Ann and Ken are a good example of a couple whose marriage survived because they were aware of conflicts and willing to deal with them. Good marriages are not devoid of conflict, pain, and disappointment. Healthy marriages are characterized by sharing both happy and sad experiences, a commitment to dealing with individual and couple issues, and the ability to grow as people and as a couple.

CLOSING THOUGHTS

The equity model of marriage involves freedom for individual development while maintaining cohesiveness and intimacy. Both partners are aware of the stresses and tensions that occur as a result of balancing careers, children, and a changing sexual relationship. They recognize there are more similarities than differences between women and men. They value equity, respect, trust, and intimacy, and strive to nurture the couple bond. Just as important, they are committed to dealing with conflicts and reaching mutually satisfying agreements. A vital and stable marriage brings out the best in each individual, involves a positive influence process, and is based on respect, equity and trust.

6

GUIDELINES FOR YOUR MARITAL AND SEXUAL RELATIONSHIP

There are no right and wrong rules applicable to all marriages. Each couple needs to develop their unique marital and sexual style. The following guidelines are to increase awareness and facilitate intimacy. We believe in these guidelines theoretically, utilize them clinically, and apply them personally.

1. Intimacy enhances your sexual relationship.
2. The better the communication, especially the ability to make clear and direct sexual requests, the more satisfying the sex.
3. Couple time is crucial to keep your intimate relationship vital.
4. Display of affection and touching occurs in the regular course of your life, both inside and outside the bedroom.
5. Be spontaneous and playful in sensual and sexual interactions.
6. Maintain an attitude of sexual experimentation and openness.
7. Learn to laugh off, or at least not overreact to, mediocre or unsatisfying sexual experiences.
8. Both men and women can enjoy pleasuring/foreplay, intercourse, and afterplay/afterglow.
9. Understand and accept changes in sexual response and body image that come with the maturing of the relationship and the aging process.
10. Caring and commitment nurtures intimacy.

Let's consider each guidelines as specifically and explicitly as possible. Sometimes couples attempt to apply techniques that experts claim will improve their marriage, and find not only don't they help, but they are harmful. For certain marriages, a particular guideline is simply not appropriate. Often, although the intention might be good and you're using the "right" terminology, the emotional and behavioral follow-through is weak. Barry has listened with amazement to couples who claimed to be communicating honestly, but instead were defensive and manipulative; couples who said they argued well, but were intimidating and hitting below the belt; couples who supposedly had fun were having a dull time doing something neither really wanted to because it was the "in" thing; couples who boasted of open, experimental, and playful sexual interactions, but one partner made demands and coerced the other to engage in stimulation she didn't enjoy.

These guidelines reflect complex attitudes and skills that require practice, clear and constructive feedback, and refinement before they become a comfortable part of your couple style. Making a New Year's resolution to change is not enough. Thoughtfulness, psychological energy, practice, and constructive feedback are required as well as the commitment to successfully implement these guidelines.

Guideline 1. Intimacy enhances your sexual relationship. There is an age-old theoretical argument, "Can you have sex without love?" Of course you can. People can be sexually functional in nonloving relationships; the scientific data on that question is clear. However, psychologists believe sexuality is most satisfying in the context of an intimate, committed relationship. Emotional intimacy involves revealing yourself to the spouse—not only loving feelings and positive characteristics, but personal weaknesses and doubts. In an intimate marriage, you have the freedom to disclose vulnerabilities and are still loved and accepted. You don't need to maintain secrets or worry that if the spouse discovers them she will not respect or love you. Intimacy means sharing happy, loving feelings as well as problems, disappointments, and angry feelings. These are dealt with in the context of an intimate, secure marriage. You trust the spouse not to abuse your disclosures, to support you through bad times, and to accept vulnerable and problem areas. The spouse respects and loves you for who you really are, not the public image you project.

Sexually, you enjoy giving and receiving pleasure *with* each other rather than performing *for* each other. If she is not lubricated or he does not have an erection, the partners will not berate each other but accept this as a bad time for intercourse. You could engage in sensual touching or an erotic nonintercourse scenario. Your couple style allows both partners to initiate and request sensual and sexual activities. If you want to be the receiver of cunnilingus or fellatio and not have to reciprocate this time, the spouse can enjoy giving pleasure without saying, ''You owe me one.'' Intimacy is *not* idealized, romantic, problem-free sexuality. Being intimate includes giving and receiving negative feedback and dealing with emotional and sexual problems. It means being responsive when she requests he express what he's feeling just before orgasm. It means he is free to tell her to stroke his penis with a firm and fast rhythm. Intimacy involves sharing sexual desires, feelings, and requests as you experience them. This is the key to creative, intimate sexuality.

Guideline 2. The better the communication, especially the ability to make clear and direct sexual requests, the more satisfying the sex. Communication is one of the most crucially important and yet one of the most poorly used concepts in human behavior. We advocate personal, clear, direct, high-quality communication. This is very different from the general, ambiguous, indirect, and low-quality communication which is the norm. It is the difference between saying, ''What would you like to do?'' or ''I need you to massage me just the way I tell you or I won't get turned on,'' and saying, ''I like the way you're stroking me, but it would be better if you moved your hand about an inch and touched in a gentle, more tender way.'' Communication can and should be both verbal and nonverbal. The ability to guide the partner by putting your hand over his and showing where and how you wish to be touched is an important skill. This ''hand override'' technique is very effective. Another nonverbal guiding technique is to take the partner's hand or head and move it to the area you want him to stimulate.

There's a crucial difference between a request and a demand. A request is *asking* something from the spouse. Disclose your feelings and what you want. Maintain a concern for her perceptions, feelings, and preferences. The partner can accept the request, modify it, or reject it. A demand says she must do it now, do it your way, or there will be consequences. Requests result in sharing pleasure, demands result in feelings of anger, resentment, and pressure to meet performance requirements. Requests enhance the couple bond. Demands allow you to get what you want at the moment, but cause a breach in communication and intimacy. Requests broaden opportunities for emotional and sexual intimacy.

Guideline 3. Couple time is crucial to keep your intimate relationship vital. This is a crucial guideline. We, like many couples, live hectic lives with demands on our time from children and a grandchild, careers, household chores, friends, extended family, and community activities. Couple time receives a high priority; it is jealously guarded.

Couple time might consist of a fifteen-minute chat on the porch, drinking tea, sharing experiences and feelings about the week; dinner together, without kids or friends, and then a long walk; a weekend trip to the city—as a couple, not a family. Before doing separate chores during the evening, make a date to meet later over a drink and discuss what you've been doing, chat about the next day, or engage in nondemand pleasuring which may or may not proceed to intercourse. It is easy to take the spouse for granted and allow the couple bond to erode.

Couples claim they have time together because they see each other coming and going. The couple time we're advocating is quality, interactive time. It involves touching and talking where you connect emotionally and feel caring and cared about.

Couple time includes the period before and after intercourse. Having a relaxing bath—during which the spouse has come in and out of the bathroom talking and teasing—and, as you dry off, receiving an invitation to come to bed, can be exciting. Afterplay is a particularly good time for feeling close and being together. After sharing sex, it is natural to share feelings about you and the relationship. People are more emotionally open before and after a sexual experience.

Guideline 4. Affection and touching occurs in the regular course of your life, both inside and outside the bedroom. Pleasure and affection belong in your life, not just in the bedroom when the lights are out, the kids asleep, and his penis is in her vagina. Many couples feel they have outgrown the stage where they hold hands and really kiss (not a perfunctory peck).

That's a destructive myth; you never outgrow the need for touching and affection. Maintaining affectionate contact as a regular part of your life allows sexual feelings to flow naturally rather than isolating sex as an activity unto itself, separate from the rest of your life and relationship. It's fun to stimulate the partner's breast as she's bending over to kiss you good-bye on her way to work. These pleasant images linger throughout the day and make it more likely you'll feel sexual in the evening.

A hug and kiss while paying bills is comforting. Having contact and support while doing one of life's most odious tasks makes it more livable. Being affectionate while watching TV with the kids in the family room can be good for both you and the children. Seeing parents touching, hugging, and kissing is a good model for children. We are not suggesting being sensual or sexual in front of the children—that is a private activity. Being affectionate in front of children and family hugs are a positive part of sexuality education. Integrating touching and affection, whether in the kitchen or bedroom, in your car or walking in public, as a couple or in front of the children—is an affirmation of caring and a source of sexual desire. Sexuality is more than genitals, intercourse, and the few seconds of orgasm. Sexuality is a way of expressing warmth, affection, attraction, connection, and desire.

Guideline 5. Be spontaneous and playful in sensual and sexual interactions. Sex is special when it's tender and warm, extending over a two-hour period. It can have all the romance of a candlelight dinner with wine, lobster, and intercourse as dessert. However, if that were the format for each experience, sex would become dull. It's nice to spice up life with a "quickie" or stand-up intercourse; sometimes you need tuna salad or hamburger so you can appreciate veal. When you're in touch with desires and feelings, sex is spontaneous and creative. Planned, romantic sex can be as satisfying as unplanned, spontaneous sex. Sometimes sex can be intense and passionate, other times tender and sensuous. Waking up before the partner and waking him by sucking on his penis is arousing, but so can being warm, slow, and sensuous. The key is to be aware of your feelings in the moment and open to the spouse's desires.

Sexual arousal can arise from being silly and playful. For example, while playing cards and joking, you have a simulated fight with a resulting desire for sex. If you're usually task-oriented in the morning, on a whim go back to bed after breakfast. After a hard game of tennis, take a shower and engage in a second game—of sex! Being turned on need not always result in intercourse. Enjoy the playful or erotic moment for itself. Those times it does lead to intercourse are all the better.

Guideline 6. Maintain an attitude of sexual experimentation and openness. If you believe you know all there is to know about each other and there is no need for experimentation, this becomes a self-fulfilling prophecy. Sex becomes dull, routine, and stagnant. You feel the only way to spice up sex is to have an affair. When your attitude is one of experimentation and openness, then it too becomes a self-fulfilling prophecy. Marital sex continues to evolve and remain vital.

We have been married thirty-one years, and never cease to be amazed at new sexual awareness about ourselves, each other, and how we share pleasure. In large part this comes from our conscious commitment to experiment and share. When first married, we believed the hard task would be to develop an open, free sexual style. What we have come to understand is that the real challenge is to commit the time and energy to maintain a vital intimate bond.

We set aside time for an extended sexual session every six weeks or so. The focus is experimenting with something new. It might be simple, such as using a new body lotion or trying a variation of an intercourse position. Other times we do something more elaborate, like going to an old inn and, after a candlelight dinner, making love on an eighteenth-century couch. Or we would drop the children at a baby-sitter and return home, take the phone off the hook, and have a three-hour love session in the family room in front of the fireplace while listening to a new tape. Other couples use techniques such as pretending they're on a first date and engaging in the coy give-and-take of the sexual seduction game. What fits your feelings and needs? Attitude is key—awareness of and desire to experiment, learn, and grow. You care enough about the marriage and marital sex to keep it vital and satisfying.

Guideline 7. Learn to laugh off, or at least not overreact to, mediocre or unsatisfying sexual experiences. An oppressive new sex myth is that all sexual experiences should be fully functional and equally arousing for both partners. Otherwise, according to this myth, you have a sexual dysfunction or hang-up. In reality, couples who feel a high level of sexual satisfaction report 40 percent of sexual experiences are very satisfactory for both partners; in 25–30 percent one partner finds it very fulfilling, while the other finds it enjoyable; 20–25 percent of sexual interactions are moderately satisfying for one partner, the other goes along for the ride (although enjoying the response of the spouse); and in 5 to 10 percent of sexual interactions, sex is either mediocre or unsuccessful. This happens with us, as it does to other couples. Somewhere in the middle of pleasuring or even during intercourse, one of us—usually Barry—will ask if the other is "into it." If the response is, "No, but I thought you were," we'll laugh it off and say, "Let's be sexual tomorrow." We try to get together during the next day or two when we're awake, receptive and responsive, so thoughts of the unsatisfying sex don't linger.

Many couples overreact to a poor sexual experience and either don't talk or endlessly discuss the problem and whose fault it was. If mediocre or dysfunctional sex is a frequent occurrence, you need to discuss your couple sexual style in an open, frank manner, and consider whether you would benefit from couples sex therapy. However, if problems are infrequent, accept the fact that sexual response is variable and don't turn it into a major issue. To use a cliché, "Don't make a mountain out of a molehill." Mediocre, uninteresting, or failed sexual experiences are not only to be expected, but are a natural aspect of your humanness and variability as a couple. You don't always cook a perfect dinner or have a wonderful time at a party, nor do your children always behave perfectly. It is unrealistic to expect sex to always be functional and satisfying. There is a next time, and that time will be easier if this time you can laugh and be accepting.

Guideline 8. Both men and women can enjoy pleasuring/ foreplay, intercourse, and afterplay/afterglow. Many people consider pleasuring/foreplay to be primarily or exclusively for getting the woman ready for intercourse. A "sophisticated" man considers foreplay not a duty but a mark of concern for his wife and a measure of his expertise as a lover. The idea a man can enjoy sensuality and pleasuring for himself strikes him as unmasculine. Intercourse is viewed as the domain of the male, although there is pressure on women to have an orgasm during intercourse. Of course, once a man ejaculates, sex is over. These rigid sexual perceptions cause miscommunication and resentment. They build performance anxiety, reduce pleasure, and interfere with feeling like an intimate team.

Pleasuring/foreplay, intercourse, and afterplay/afterglow are integral expressions of sexuality rather than arbitrary components in which the male takes one role and the female another. Pleasure is open to both partners throughout the sexual experience. Female sexual response is more *complex* and *variable* than male response. For women, arousal takes longer and requires more time setting the mood, engaging in pleasuring, and building eroticism. The woman might be nonorgasmic, singly orgasmic, or multiorgasmic, which can occur during pleasuring, intercourse, or afterplay. The male typically has one orgasm occurring during intercourse. Female sexual response is different, not better or worse, than male response. Sexuality is a matter of pleasure and mutuality, not performance and competition.

Both can enjoy pleasuring. This is unlikely if the man "does the woman" for twenty minutes with the goal of arousing her for intercourse. Sex is more involving and arousing if there is mutual pleasuring. Sexuality is more satisfying when you are open to giving and receiving pleasure-oriented touching. The male can enjoy slow, teasing arousal during which his erection will wax and wane. He is open to receiving as well as giving pleasure. This slow, interactive pleasuring scenario results in more satisfying intercourse and orgasm.

As you share pleasure in the process of mutual arousal and stop seeing it as work toward a goal, intercourse is viewed as a natural extension of pleasuring. Sex is not an act in which the male must respond with an erection and the female must respond with an orgasm. Some women are orgasmic with intercourse. Most women enjoy intercourse, but find it easier and more pleasurable to be orgasmic with manual, oral, or rubbing stimulation. This is a matter of couple style and preference, not a question of a "right" or "wrong" way to have an orgasm. Intercourse is an intimate sharing and coming together. It is not necessary for the woman to be orgasmic during intercourse to meet his expectations or prove something to herself or anyone else. Intercourse will be more satisfying for both people if they focus on pleasure and arousal, not performance. Intercourse is best viewed as a natural extension of the pleasuring process, not apart from that process.

The afterplay/afterglow phase is not just tacked on; it is integral to lovemaking. Physiologically, you just shared an intense experience. Your body is gradually returning to the unstimulated state. Psychologically, this is an excellent time to share feelings and closeness. Some couples enjoy lying together and holding; others drink a glass of wine and talk; still others engage in a playful pillow fight. The important thing is nurturing your intimate bond.

Guideline 9. Understand and accept changes in sexual response and body image that come with the maturing of the relationship and the aging process. Our bodies change gradually in both appearance and function as we age. Aging does *not* mean becoming nonsexual, unless you fall into the trap of narrowly defining sexuality by youth, beauty, and rapid response. Partners who view sexuality as pleasure oriented, who realize arousal comes from sharing and stimulation, and who enjoy the receptivity and responsivity of the partner, find sex satisfying as they age. The changes that occur with aging are gradual, not dramatic. Aging alters sexual functioning, but does not end it. You are a sexual person from the day you're born to the day you die.

Self-image and sexual response are influenced by how you treat yourself. If you gain weight, do not exercise, smoke, drink to excess, and do not attend to your body, you will be less healthy and feel less sexual. People who take care of their bodies, have regular sleep patterns, eat well, exercise, do not smoke, and drink moderately are more likely to be healthy and sexually responsive.

As you age, sexual arousal is slower, and frequency lessens. However, the enjoyment of being together and experiencing pleasure, arousal, and orgasm is very much alive. Men no longer function automatically and autonomously, which can be an advantage. Intimate, interactive sexuality is superior to automatic arousal and erections. Youthful sex is like a wild, exciting ride over unexplored rapids, with excitement from the sense of adventure and conquest. Mature sex is like skillfully canoeing a scenic river. You can enjoy and savor its changing moods and seasons. The couple who accept their aging as a natural evolution and not a tragic event have a healthy attitude that will deliver continual sexual dividends.

Guideline 10. Caring and commitment nurtures your intimate bond. When a couple begins dating, they experience romantic ecstasy. There is novelty, excitement about what will develop, willingness to overcome barriers in order to be with the lover. Some feel it is tragic that romantic ecstasy does not last. We believe it is a good thing. Marriage cannot be based on novelty, ecstasy, and conquest. Seeking a perpetual return to these states is self-defeating, leading to frustration. Going backward only works in the movies. Emotional and sexual intimacy form a mature, solid, and secure basis for marital sex. It is possible, and indeed critical, to grow as people while maintaining a commitment to the marital bond. Changing involves an integration of the old and new. You change as you age. Be aware of personal, physical, and sexual changes and integrate them into your intimate relationship.

When you read about an oral sex technique you'd like to experiment with, request it in a caring way, refrain from being demanding. Your style of adapting the oral sex experience will be different from that described in an article or seen in a movie. Don't worry about keeping up with new sexual trends. Be aware of your experiences and preferences. Choose how to integrate new techniques and scenarios into your lovemaking.

Growing entails an attitude that you invite change rather than stagnate. These changes are integrated into your lovemaking style. In marriage, there will be periods of stress, frustration, and discomfort. There also will also be periods of joy, discovery, and pride. Dealing with a difficult situation and resolving a problem strengthens the couple bond. Coping with problems is a stressful, but necessary, growing experience. Sharing sad as well as joyful experiences increases intimacy. A satisfying, intimate, and secure marriage involves being open to sexual and emotional growth, dealing with the good and the bad.

CLOSING THOUGHTS

These guidelines are to help you think and talk about intimacy and sexuality. They are not hard-and-fast rules. Implement these guidelines so they enhance your marital and sexual style. The guidelines emphasize positive attitudes even more than specific behaviors. You owe it yourselves and your marriage to grow as individuals and as a couple.

7

SEXUAL VARIATIONS—WHEN DOES EXPERIMENTATION BECOME KINKY?

Variety and experimentation are catchwords used in the media as well as by sex therapists. But what does this mean? Learning to be comfortable with giving and receiving oral sex? Becoming involved in swinging and group ambisexuality? If we as a couple choose to experiment sexually and challenge inhibited patterns, do we have to go all the way and try everything we've heard or read about? Do we need to *prove* we're liberated?

Variety and experimentation are healthy for marital sexuality. We encourage couples to experiment with a range of sexual scenarios and techniques. However, experimentation should *not* be to prove anything to anyone, nor involve performance demands, nor be manipulative or coercive. Experimentation is to increase sharing, pleasure and eroticism. As long as the focus is on pleasure not performance, on requests rather than demands, on honesty not manipulation, experimentation will enhance sexuality. If you approach this as mutual exploration you will not feel disappointed or intimidated. You are not on a search for a goal, but on a journey to enjoy the sexual discovery process. Be open to experiences that enhance eroticism and satisfaction.

Before setting out on this journey, allow us to offer a warning: don't fall into the new, sexually sophisticated trap of having to prove you are sexually liberated. The notion that you "should" desire each new technique—whether anal stimulation, being sexual in a hot tub, masturbating in front of the partner, watching X-rated videos, making love standing up, or playing out group sex fantasies—is just another form of sexual fascism. Sexual comfort and freedom means accepting your preferences and choices. Couples who feel they must try each sexual technique in order to prove they are not inhibited are in a worse position than sexually repressed couples. With this in mind, let us examine a range of sexual variations, scenarios, and techniques.

ORAL SEX

The mouth and genitals are the two most pleasure-giving and pleasure-receiving parts of the human body. Traditionally, oral-genital sex has been viewed as exotic and exciting, but also anxiety-provoking and guilt-inducing. Oral sex is not only normal but one of the most intimate, pleasurable, and satisfying means of expressing yourself with the person you love. As with any sexual technique, there are individual differences and preferences. Individuals or couples who choose not to engage in or who do not enjoy oral-genital stimulation are normal, not sexually repressed. It is your right and choice not to include oral sex in your repertoire.

It is interesting but baffling why so much of oral sex (cunnilingus and fellatio) is shrouded in a cloud of dirtiness, or at least naughtiness. Slang terms such as "go down on," "69", "blow job," "eat her out," and "suck him off" have negative, aggressive connotations. In pornographic magazines and X-rated movies, there is an inordinate emphasis on oral-genital sex, with special emphasis on domination and humiliation. The subtle, and not so subtle, message was oral sex is exciting but degrading, an act of lust rather than sharing intimacy and passion. The message was oral sex is primarily for men. The woman's role is to pretend she enjoys it. The chauvinist joke is men are on the lookout for a woman who is willing to let him ejaculate in her mouth (and swallow his semen), but she's perverted if she does.

The truth is oral sex is pleasurable and loving, an intimate sharing without connotations of dominance or humiliation. You can enjoy high levels of arousal and lusty feelings without concern that you're being perverse or animalistic. Both women and men enjoy giving and receiving oral stimulation.

What are the best oral sex techniques? Is it okay if he ejaculates in her mouth? What if she passes gas while he's orally stimulating her? Is it okay if he thrusts his pelvis or should he be passive? Why does she feel self-conscious when he's lying between her legs? Why is it easier for her to be multiorgasmic during cunnilingus? Is mutual oral sex ("69") better than taking turns? Is the taste of vaginal secretions bad for his breath? These are among the questions couples have, but are too embarrassed to ask. There is not one best technique nor one right way to engage in oral sex. We encourage you to experiment, share, and choose based on your preferences and style.

The best way to approach oral-genital sex is comfortably. Oral sex can involve kissing, licking, sucking, biting. Start by doing oral stimulation on other body parts—neck, back, breasts, face—before moving to the genitals. Try stimulation with one partner giving before trying mutual oral stimulation. Instead of pressing for orgasm, focus on oral pleasuring. Explore, see what feels good and what the partner enjoys. Most people are not responsive to oral stimulation unless they are moderately aroused. He might run his tongue around her vulva before doing a rapid sucking motion focused on the labia and clitoral area. Oral stimulation, like manual and intercourse stimulation, progresses from slow, tender touching. This allows the arousal process to gradually build.

For many women, oral stimulation is the easiest and fastest way to achieve orgasm. More women experience multiorgasmic response with cunnilingus than any other technique. Although males feel highly aroused through oral stimulation, they may be embarrassed or self-conscious asking for or guiding the partner in what is most erotic. The woman feels confused because she experiences pressure to orally stimulate his penis, but has no guidance or feedback. As is true of other sexual techniques, oral sex does not come naturally. Even basics, such as putting the penis to the side of the mouth so it doesn't cause a gag reflex or holding your hand on his penis while he thrusts, need to be communicated and practiced. Start oral stimulation by kissing or licking around the shaft of the penis before putting it in your mouth. Do what's comfortable—stimulating the glans with your tongue, sucking with your lips closed, moving your tongue when the penis is in your mouth—before asking what's best for him. Most males want the woman to be harder and more forceful in doing fellatio, but are shy about requesting this.

The question of ejaculation is one of the most emotionally loaded and individualistic preferences. Does he want to? Some men prefer oral sex for arousal and ejaculate during intercourse. Others not only want to ejaculate, but see it as symbolic that she swallow the semen. Semen is germfree, safe, and even low caloric. Many women do not like semen gushing into their mouths. They enjoy sucking and licking the penis, but not ejaculation. The couple has to establish, in a non-coercive manner, a style of oral sex that enhances comfort, pleasure, and eroticism for each. The most common pattern is to use fellatio as a pleasuring technique and then switch to intercourse. When fellatio is pursued to orgasm, some males withdraw right before ejaculation, others ejaculate in her mouth. Some women prefer spitting the semen out, other prefer swallowing.

WEEKENDS AWAY

Are parents selfish, hedonistic people if they enjoy weekends away without children? Is your life an endless seeking of excitement without attending to responsibilities and caring for children? Should you feel guilty about taking time for yourselves as a couple, especially when sexual sharing is a major component?

We believe weekends away without children is one of the best things you can do for yourself and the marriage. The central relationship in a family is the husband-wife bond. As long as this remains strong, it is easier to deal with career, financial, extended family, home, and parenting issues. We try to have at least one and preferably two weekends a year to ourselves to reenergize our intimate bond.

Sex is not the most important aspect of marriage, but is integral to the couple bond. Sexuality has three important functions—sharing pleasure, reducing tension, and reinforcing intimacy. A weekend away gives you the time and privacy to be an intimate couple. The strengthened couple bond allows you to function better as a person and a parent.

When our children were younger, we traded baby-sitting with other families and watched their children when they took a weekend away. The children looked forward to this because it gave them a chance to have friends spend a weekend. Believe it or not, it's not that much harder to watch six rather than three children; they entertain and enjoy each other.

The weekend need not be focused on sex. You can enjoy

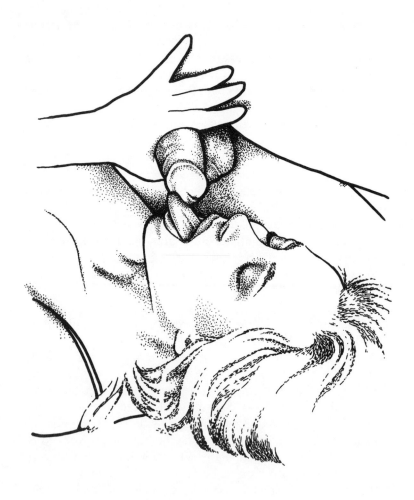

The mouth and genitals are the most pleasure-giving and plea-sure-receiving parts of the human body. Oral sex is intimate, pleasurable and erotic for the giver and the receiver.

skiing, sailing, seeing a play, antiquing, reading a book, sight-seeing, and going to dinner. However, do not overschedule. Be sure you have time for each other, to talk and for leisurely sex. Being together, holding hands, and touching builds a sensual mood. Weekends away allow experimentation with sex in the morning, afternoon, or early evening. Break out of "sex as the last thing at night after everything else is taken care of" routine.

It is important to have weekends away when children are young. The parent of a young child knows how easy it is for children to dominate every waking moment. What is less apparent is the need for weekends when children are older, especially during adolescence. Adolescence can be a tumultuous and difficult time. Not surprisingly, one of the most stressful periods in adult life is parenting adolescents. You need a weekend away to reenergize you and your marital bond. It helps prepare you for the stage of being a couple again, when children leave home.

One of our favorite scenarios was to return to our house and spend a weekend at home alone. Whatever you do and however you as a couple decide to do it, a weekend or even a night away can revitalize you, the relationship, and sexuality. It can be a creative, fun time. Ideas for this book were developed on a weekend away.

SENSUALITY AND PLEASURING

Whoever heard of a married couple being playful, sexually turned on, and not proceeding to intercourse? Being nude and having a sensual body massage just to enjoy the experience? A perversion? No, it is a way to keep in touch with your sensuality and sexuality. Reaffirm sexuality as a means of sharing pleasure and intimacy, not a command performance. Touching and being sexual without the demand that it culminate in intercourse each time is one of the best ways to keep a relationship fresh and spontaneous. It has the beneficial side effect of increasing intercourse frequency. Since you maintain physical connection, when one or the other feels desirous, the transition from touching to intercourse is easier.

We set aside an evening every six weeks to engage in non-demand pleasuring, agreeing beforehand this will *not* end in intercourse. Sometimes the evening is a relaxing one during which we lie around, drink wine, and listen to music. Touching is gentle and sensuous, but not erotic. Other times sexual arousal builds. Teasing touching and sensuality increases anticipation and results in erotic feelings that may proceed to orgasm for one or both, depending on feelings and desires.

Pleasuring brings back memories of teenage years, when petting and necking were particularly exciting, before engaging in the "real thing." Couples have the attitude that since intercourse is available, enjoying anticipation, unpredictability, and variable arousal is not acceptable. Touching that does not proceed to intercourse is derogatorily labeled "immature" or "sexual teasing." What nonsense. This attitude is a major reason for mechanical, routine, and unsatisfying marital sex. Youthful sex was filled with a sense of adventure, exploration, and playfulness. It is easy to fall into the trap of touching always leading to intercourse. Pleasuring adds excitement, variety, a sense of exploration, spontaneity, and unpredictability. Sensuality is a prime source of sexual desire.

MASTURBATION

Did you know that over half of married women and two thirds of married men occasionally masturbate? The old view was that masturbation is a form of self-abuse which causes physical and psychological problems, from acne to social isolation. A recent, more enlightened view was that masturbation is a developmental phase that young men—but not women—experience, which ceases after they begin intercourse.

Research and clinical practice indicates that masturbation is the best way for a man or woman to learn about his/her body, sexual responsivity, and orgasm. Both men and women masturbate before marriage, and both masturbate after marriage. In fact, rates of female masturbation increase after marriage.

For the married person, masturbation can serve many functions. It can be a way of dealing with sexual desires when the spouse is away or ill; provide a mechanism to keep in touch with your sexuality; an orgasmic outlet when there is a discrepancy in partners' sex drives; a vehicle to experiment with a new erotic technique or fantasy. Of course, as with all aspects of sexuality, masturbation can be misused. Masturbation can be employed as a weapon to make the spouse uncomfortable, a compulsive behavior to deal with boredom or anxiety, a way to avoid dealing with sexual dissatisfaction, or a means of keeping emotional and sexual distance.

One exercise employed in sex therapy is masturbation in front of the partner. This can be arousing, especially for the person observing. It provides an excellent way to teach the partner how you like to be touched and your pattern of arousal. Consider whether this form of experimentation would be worthwhile for you.

DIFFERENT SETTINGS AND TIMES

For most couples, sex = the bedroom late at night. Couples say sex is important, but it is given the last priority—late at night, when all other important and unimportant chores have been completed. What about setting a special time and place for a sexual encounter? Physiologically, the best time for sex is in the morning. Your body is rested, sleep and dreams have rested your mind, and testosterone levels are highest in the morning. On weekends, rather than jumping out of bed to start chores or getting the paper and busily informing yourself of the world's woes, why not take time to be sensual and/or sexual? Waking to a gentle massage, having your breasts fondled or penis stroked, is better than a cup of coffee. You might like a "quickie" intercourse before leaving for work. You could carry pleasant memories during the day, anticipating a romantic and mutually involving evening.

What about nooners? Instead of a business lunch at which you eat too much, drink too much, and spend too much money come home and add a little sexual pleasure to your day. During the weekend, ask neighbors to watch your children or get the kids involved in an activity so you can go upstairs, lock the door, take the phone off the hook, and enjoy yourselves.

What about sex before dinner or early in the evening? Exercise—including sex—before eating improves digestive processes. If you can't sleep or wake early, what about waking the partner by fondling and caressing? Nothing is more inviting than waking up and realizing the partner is aroused and desires you.

What would it be like to make love in the kitchen? On the

rug in front of the fireplace? What about a deserted beach? In
the back seat of the car like you did twenty years ago? Of course,
the bedroom is more convenient and comfortable, but wouldn't
you occasionally like to be adventuresome and take a risk? Even
more intriguing, what about going to your office at night or on
a weekend when no one is there? You could have sex in the
office chair, on the rug, or even on the desk—pleasant memories
for when you're stuck in a boring meeting. In suggesting these,
we don't want you to feel pressured to do any or all, but consider
whether you want to try one or two on for size and see if it fits
your erotic needs.

SEXUAL FANTASIES

Sexual fantasies are the most flexible and adaptable aphrodis-
iacs. People use fantasies during masturbation and feel fine about
it. However, people feel strange using fantasies when having sex
with their spouse. Does it mean she wants to be with another
man or he wants group sex?

The great majority of us have unusual and even bizarre sexual
fantasies, at least occasionally. You might fantasize about forced
sex or being forced, others watching and admiring your performance, five people making love to you at the same time, a
ménage-a-trois with the spouse and your business partner. These
fantasies are hard to accept, but the hardest of all, although the
most frequent, are fantasies about another partner. Whether it's
the next-door neighbor, the person at the drugstore, the spouse's
best friend, an attractive individual you see on the bus, or a
movie star, you feel anxious and guilty. This is especially true
when you're fantasizing about another person during intercourse
with your spouse.

Having and enjoying a fantasy is not the same as desiring to
actually experience the behavior. Most of us would not like,
much less participate in, the sex fantasies we use. What gives
fantasies special power is they are illicit, have socially unacceptable themes, and rebel against societal norms. It is one thing
to be aroused by the image; it is altogether different to act out
the behavior.

Most fantasies are best kept as fantasies. When people do act
them out, they are usually disappointed and get into situations

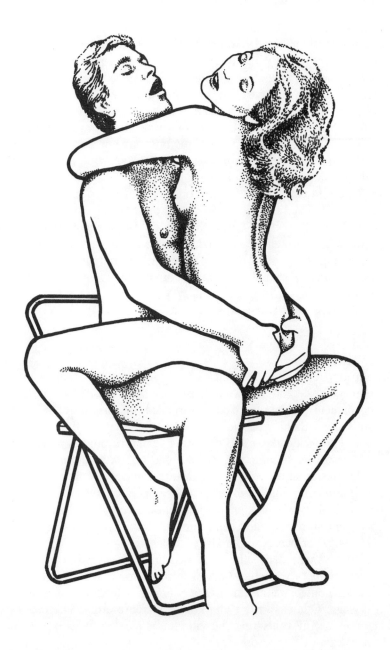

Intercourse in the sitting position allows you to experience alternate ways of making love.

with negative consequences. Fantasizing about sex with another person is natural and harmless. Don't view it as a sign of unfaithfulness or not wanting to make love with your intimate partner. You are having sex with each other and enjoying it—including the fantasies. The role of fantasy is to spice up your sex life. Fantasies are best thought of as an erotic technique that builds bridges to sexual desire and arousal. Fantasies only get you into trouble when they become obsessive or associated with guilt. Give yourself permission to use a range of fantasies to enhance desire and eroticism.

The following techniques are ones we ourselves choose not to engage in, but this is a question of preference. Don't judge a technique as "normal" or "abnormal." As long as both of you agree to experiment, don't feel coerced, are not trying to prove something, and it isn't done in a harmful or compulsive manner, it is a normal sexual variation. You might choose to do this experimentally or just occasionally, or it may become an important part of your couple sexual style.

VIBRATORS

In our technological society, where everything is being done by machines, shouldn't we at least keep sex natural? Do we need mechanical gadgets to make us aroused and orgasmic? No, we don't *need* them, but many couples find that a vibrator adds variety to lovemaking and enhances sexual responsiveness.

Vibrators first came into widespread use as an adjunct to female masturbation. There are different types of vibrators, the most popular being hand-held, battery-operated, two-speed models with two to four attachments. They are sold in drug or department stores as hand, face, or back massagers as well as in sex shops, or can be ordered by mail.

Couples who derive the most pleasure from vibrators use them as an adjunct to touching, not as a magic toy that substitutes for partner contact. You can use a vibrator to enhance a sensual massage. Others use the vibrator to increase arousal before intercourse. Still others use the vibrator as part of sex play to help the woman achieve orgasm. Some couples use vibrator stimulation during intercourse to increase clitoral stimulation, which allows the woman to be orgasmic during coitus. The vibrator is not just the woman's device; men can enjoy giving and receiving vibrator stimulation.

Some uses of the vibrator might appeal to you; others might strike you as strange or "kinky." Our message is not that you have to try it, it's an option to enhance sexual pleasure and arousal.

ANAL INTERCOURSE

People associate the anus with dirtiness. What people do not realize is the anal area contains a large number of nerve endings. The anal area is an erogenous zone just as is the mons and labia or the shaft of the penis and testicles. Some people express a good deal of interest in and arousal from having their buttocks touched and stroked. Many couples enjoy rear-entry penis-vagina intercourse. Both men and women can enjoy manual stimulation around the perineum and anal area. Many couples engage in buttock and anal stimulation.

When people think of anal sex, they are specifically referring to anal intercourse. About one in four couples had experimented with anal intercourse until they were deterred by the fear of HIV/ AIDS. Being passive in anal intercourse is the most dangerous behavior for the transmission of the HIV virus. We strongly urge couples to refrain from anal intercourse, even with condoms, unless they are sure both are HIV negative.

There are many myths about anal intercourse; the most prominent being that it is a sign of "latent homosexuality." That term is probably the most misused of any in sexual language. The concept of latent homosexuality is used as a club to keep couples from experimenting because they fear this will unleash perverse tendencies. In truth, there is no such thing as an exclusive homosexual behavior. Gay couples interact sexually the same way as heterosexual couples. What makes sex homosexual is that it is engaged in by two people of the *same* sex, not the sexual behavior itself.

Anal intercourse is prepared for by using a lubricant to facilitate entry. Since the anal sphincter muscle does not easily dilate, entry should be slow and guided by the woman so she does not experience pain. Couples report discomfort on the first few insertions, but as they communicate and develop a comfortable style of insertion, the problem dissipates. One advantage of anal intercourse is the male can simultaneously provide hand stimulation of the vulva and clitoral area. Many couples enjoy anal intercourse. A major warning is not to switch from anal to vaginal intercourse because bacteria from the anus can infect the vagina. The man can use a lubricated condom during anal intercourse and remove it for vaginal intercourse. Or he could wash his penis before engaging in vaginal intercourse. This same guideline applies to manual stimulation inside the anus; wash your hands before doing vaginal stimulation.

Many couples find manual stimulation of the buttocks, perineum, and anal area more pleasurable than actual insertion. It has all the advantages of stimulating the nerve endings and providing different sensations with none of the problems of insertion. Manual anal stimulation is usually done in the context of other sexual activity, such as intercourse, breast, or penile stimulation. Anal stimulation can be a pleasurable activity, adding to the totality of the sexual encounter.

USE OF SEXUALLY EXPLICIT MATERIALS (EROTICA)

What is the difference between R-rated and XXX-rated videos? It is the difference between a romantic yet explicit presentation of sex and a nonrelational and sometimes violent or degrading presentation of the sexual encounter. Whether on a video, photos, cybersex, or a novel, the purpose is to break down inhibitions and excite you by portraying lustful, "anything goes" scenarios. Like fantasies, the techniques depicted might not be what you want to do, but watching or reading can be highly arousing.

Sharing sexually explicit material can be a couple activity, instead of the man going to a stag party and/or sneaking magazines to the office. Many couples become excited by watching a video or looking at pictures. Illicit feelings add to arousal. Erotica can be stimulating for both women and men. The VCR has revolutionized the use of erotica because people no longer have to go to distinctly unsavory XXX-rated movie houses. Erotica, X-rated videos, novels, magazines, or pictures can be shared in the privacy of your home.

A problem with pornographic materials is that they present an aggressive, male dominant, performance-oriented, and degrading view of sex. Men always have super-large erections and have orgasm after orgasm. Women always have big breasts and appear to relish the painful and acrobatic aspects of the encounter. Sex is impersonal but always perfectly performed. The message is, "The best sex is dirty sex." Isn't this opposed to what we've written concerning intimacy and pleasuring? Of course it is— yet isn't there something exciting about occasionally having a quick "fuck" or fantasizing a sexual encounter with a stranger? Looking at or reading erotica is a way to experience vicariously a wide variety of sexually stimulating situations without feeling guilt. Choose erotica that is arousing for both partners. Avoid erotica that intimidates or turns off either partner.

GROUP SEX

Radical sexual theorists believe the epitome of sexual liberation is group ambisexuality (the ability to engage in same-sex, opposite-sex, and solo-sex activity in a group setting). We believe finding the ultimate sexual behavior to prove you're liberated is a new form of sexual fascism.

Group sex is a variant some couples choose to experiment with. It has the potential to be erotic and exciting, but is often destructive. Group sex should be undertaken only after carefully discussing your feelings and motivations as well as agreeing on a plan to bail out of the experiment if it becomes destructive. In this age of STDs and HIV/AIDS, it is crucial to know the health status of people you engage with sexually and utilize safe-sex techniques.

There are many varieties of group sex, including organized swinging (either open to observation or done privately), bisexual group encounters, simultaneous group sex featuring "daisy chains," and threesomes. The major enticement is to give and receive varying kinds of sexual stimulation with a variety of partners. The experience of fellating someone and at the same time having intercourse, of three people stimulating you simultaneously, or having vaginal and anal intercourse at the same time can provide a great deal of excitement. Another source of arousal is observing people having a variety of sexual interactions. Some men feel very excited watching their wife and another woman engaging in cunnilingus. A woman may become aroused when watching two women stimulating her husband. This also highlights the major psychological drawback of group sex: jealousy, performance comparisons, and a sense of alienating, impersonal sex. The major health concern is exposure to multiple partners with the ensuing danger of STDs and HIV/AIDS.

Advocates of group sex claim it is a sharing of multiple pleasures in which openness and honesty overcome jealousy. These relationships, they say, are experimental and nonmanipulative. Those who disparage group sex, including some who had previously engaged in it, see it as more attractive in theory than in practice. Couples rationalize bad feelings, but eventually one or both feel manipulated, used, jealous, and/or distrustful. The empirical data indicates group sex is destructive to most couples' marital relationship. We do not advise group sexual experimentation. For those who do engage in it, it is imperative that they protect their health, utilize safe-sex techniques, and are aware of the emotional risks to the individuals and the couple bond.

CLOSING THOUGHTS

There is a range of sexual variations and techniques that can provide excitement and revitalize your sexual relationship. We discussed several scenarios and techniques, some of which we've incorporated into our lives and others we have chosen not to use, either because they don't interest us or we feel they would negatively impact our relationship. You can decide which if any, would be erotic and enhancing for you.

The essence of creative sexuality does not lie in technique. The most genuine and satisfying aspect of marital sex is awareness of feelings, desires, and comfort in communicating these to the spouse. Sex is most creative not when it focuses on isolated techniques, but when it involves you as a person intimately aware of yourself and the spouse, sharing yourselves as sexual people.

8

CONCEPTION, CONTRACEPTION, AND INFERTILITY

One of the most emotionally complex and crucial decisions for a couple is whether to have children. Traditionally, the main function of sex was procreation. To be married without children was socially deviant.

In the last generation, conception has shifted from a cultural "should" to a choice, especially in terms of the number of children. The functions of sexuality are to serve as a shared pleasure, a means to reinforce and deepen intimacy, and a tension reducer to deal with the stresses of life and marriage. Conception is a potential function of sex, not its main function. Children are not necessary to justify sexuality or marriage. Ideally, a child would be planned and wanted, an affirmation of the couple bond and desire to be a family.

Issues surrounding conception and contraception are individualistic, value-laden, and complex. The United States has the highest premarital pregnancy rate of any developed country. One in 3 women has an unplanned premarital pregnancy. One in 4 brides is pregnant at the time of marriage or already has a child. Over 75 percent of teenage brides are pregnant.

Eighty percent of couples find it all too easy to get pregnant; their focus is using contraception to prevent unwanted pregnancies. One out of 5 couples experiences difficulty becoming pregnant, although less than 10 percent are unable to conceive.

We present guidelines for increasing awareness and decision making regarding conception, contraception, and family planning. There is not one right answer for all couples. The decision of whether to have children is individualistic and value-laden.

The traditional view was that the right choice is to have children, with the implication that deciding otherwise was a sign of immaturity, selfishness, or hostility to traditional values. Couples need to examine attitudes, feelings, values, and their life plan, and determine what is right for them. A child is at least an eighteen-year commitment—financially, practically, and most of all, emotionally. Pregnancy and child rearing is a choice, not a mandate. Whether to have a child, is one of the most important decisions a couple makes, and one of the most difficult to reverse. People, especially mothers, can switch careers, marriages, and living arrangements more easily than cease parenting.

There are few decisions in life that are as emotionally complex as whether to have children, when to have them, and how many to have. Barry has counseled competent, successful couples who have no trouble making million-dollar professional decisions, but wilt under the stress of a family planning choice.

Having a child is fundamentally an emotional decision. If couples decided only on the basis of financial, practical, and logical factors, no one would choose to have a child, and the human race would disappear. Just the opposite is happening—our planet is faced with a population explosion, especially in developing countries, that threatens to deplete the earth's resources. Population planning is one of the most important issues facing the world community.

The primary emotional reasons couples choose to have children is to experience the process of pregnancy, to participate in parenting a baby, and watching her grow into an independent person. Pregnancy, childbirth, and parenting are among life's unique and special experiences. Most married couples have children. Those individuals and couples who decide not to have a child deserve to have their choice respected and accepted. If couples carefully considered the decision, up to thirty percent might decide to remain childless. The time, as well as the financial and emotional commitment children require is truly daunting. The decision to be childless should be made not out of fear, but as a positive commitment to individual growth and being a couple. Couples without children report high levels of emotional and sexual satisfaction.

WAIT UNTIL MID-TWENTIES FOR MARRIAGE AND CHILDREN

Our principal guideline is that a couple should delay the time they marry—preferably to their mid-twenties—and wait at least two years in order to strengthen their marital bond before having a child. The average age for getting married is twenty-six for males and twenty-four for females. Approximately one in four brides is pregnant at time of marriage or already has a child. The typical couple has their first child within eighteen months of marriage. By age thirty the majority of people have a child, and many have two or more children.

Individuals would be wise to establish their autonomy and complete vocational or career training before marrying. Getting married between twenty-three and twenty-eight and beginning childbearing at twenty-five to thirty allows you to establish a stronger base for the marriage as well as family roles. This conceptualization, like other guidelines and viewpoints expressed throughout this book, is based on both empirical research and clinical data.

There are tremendous individual differences among people in experience, values, attitudes, and maturity. Only you can determine whether a guideline is valuable for your life and marriage. These guidelines provide information and a framework for discussion and, if appropriate, can be utilized for decision-making. We were married when Barry was twenty-three and Emily twenty-one (the average ages for our generation), and had our first child two years and one month later, barely within the guideline.

One of the most important tasks in the first two years of marriage is to establish expectations and roles which facilitate the development of intimacy and security. It's important that each person maintain her/his individuality; being a couple does not negate individual autonomy.

Bob and Susan

They married when Bob was twenty-five and Susan twenty-four, after knowing each other two years and living together six months. Both had just started in their chosen careers. Although they'd discussed what they wanted from marriage, it was not until they were actually married and dealing with everyday realities that their idealized and intellectualized concepts of marriage were made immediate. Intimacy was something they talked extensively about when living together, but once they were married they discovered an added dimension. Susan was wary of becoming overly dependent on Bob, yet both wanted trust, intimacy, and security. Each, in effect, was asking, "How can I be my own person yet still be an intimate, committed spouse?" They wanted to maintain individual interests and friends as well as cultivate couple friends and activities.

In the first year of marriage they experienced a surprising amount of conflict. In the heat of an argument Bob would say they should have just continued living together. Hearing this made Susan both angry and anxious. She felt angry at Bob's disparagement and anxious because she felt her security threatened. Bob's outburst was his way of asserting the traditional masculine role and distancing himself. Like most males, he claimed to need intimacy and security less than a woman. Yet when he was honest, Bob knew he married not for practical or societal reasons but out of a genuine desire to be with Susan and meet his needs for intimacy and security. He wanted a marriage in which he could be himself and safely communicate anxieties and vulnerabilities.

After unsettling arguments, they would discuss whether having a child might bring greater stability and provide a family atmosphere. Susan had taken a college course on the changing roles of women, and knew that for women in their twenties it was extremely difficult to manage a marriage, career, and children simultaneously. It was either the career or marriage that broke down. Although planned, wanted children are beneficial to a couple's relationship, the birth of a first child is a major transition, stressing the marital bond. Susan and Bob wisely decided to postpone having a child for another year. They wanted to focus on building a strong, cohesive marital bond. Although they communicated and supported one another, they had a difficult time arguing constructively and resolving conflicts. They were not enjoying social activities or couple time as much as they would like. Their sex life was becoming "the same old thing." In other words, they were falling into the traps that lurk in marriage. Susan and Bob wanted a satisfying marriage, but did not put energy into making it happen; they were allowing the relationship to slide toward mediocrity.

Susan resented being responsible for birth control. Early in the relationship Bob used condoms, but neither liked them. Susan tried an IUD, but disliked the cramping and heavy bleeding. She preferred the diaphragm, but did not like having to insert it each time they had sex and having to keep it in six hours afterwards. It was discouragement with other forms of contraception that led them to the birth control pill. Susan had no problems with the pill, but it seemed unfair that the burden for birth control was on her shoulders.

Sex is naturally exciting during the first weeks and months of a new relationship. Even though Bob ejaculated early and Susan had difficulty reaching orgasm, sex was frequent and fun. After eight months, Bob attained ejaculatory control and Susan was regularly orgasmic. This was facilitated by openly discussing sexuality and experimenting with sexual techniques, especially using slower coital thrusting and Susan showing Bob how to use two fingers to stimulate her clitoral area. Even more important, there was a sense of caring and working together.

Once the sexual relationship was functional, there was a decrease in communication and experimentation. They too fell into the trap of believing that once they could do it well, there was nothing left to learn and no reason to experiment further. Sexuality stagnates when no new energy is expended. Bob found sex routine and mechanical. Susan did not have sexual daydreams about Bob anymore, romance had disappeared, and she had to work at being orgasmic rather than it being a naturally flowing response. In trying to ascertain why pleasure had gone out of sex and what to do about it, they considered several alternatives, including sex therapy and techniques from sex manuals. They read articles in popular magazines and found themselves confused by the dogmatic, yet contradictory, advice.

Bob and Susan were having a hard time facing up to the core problem; they had allowed communicative, intimate sex to dissipate. They were no longer sharing experiences, interacting in a caring manner, being spontaneous, aware of each other's moods, and matching sexual interactions to their feelings. When they committed to revitalizing the intimate bond—being affectionate and playful *outside* the bedroom and sensuous and experimental during sex—there was a reawakening. Intimacy and pleasure were back in their marital sex.

The issues Susan and Bob faced will occur not only in the first two years, but throughout the marriage. Pleasure and sexual functioning are not resolved once and for all, but continue to arise as life circumstances and the marriage change. Even if you find sex satisfying at twenty-five, you will face new issues at thirty-five, forty-five, fifty-five, sixty-five, and seventy-five—in fact, as long as you are a sexual couple. This is not a symptom of a problematic marriage. You are changing as people, your marital relationship is changing, so your sexual relationship not only *can* change but *should*. This is equally true of your communication process, enjoyment of each other, and conflict resolution skills.

Bob and Susan were now ready to discuss children. They had couple friends who had decided to remain childless. Couples need to consider carefully whether their desire to have children is based on what is expected of them—e.g., on their parents wanting grandchildren. In the best of all worlds, a couple would not have children unless they were sure they had a viable marriage and were willing to make an eighteen-year commitment to parenting. Some couples (perhaps thirty percent) would be better to decide not to have children.

After discussing the emotional, financial, psychological, and practical pros and cons, Susan and Bob chose to have children. They were pleased they'd waited four years before trying to get pregnant. They needed that time to solidify their marital and sexual bond. Susan stopped taking birth control pills. They were happy to be among those couples for whom getting pregnant is fun and easy. It was great having sex with the intention of becoming pregnant. There is something very special about wondering if this is the time you will conceive. Trying to become pregnant is a major stimulus to sexual desire, a natural aphrodisiac.

Steve and Judy

In many ways Steve and Judy were a typical couple, marrying when Steve was twenty-six and Judy twenty-four. They decided to postpone children while Steve completed his graduate work.

Since there were few financial responsibilities, Judy decided to obtain further career training. Five years later, both were involved in their careers, doing well financially, and had the money and time for a three-week vacation and skiing weekends. Both, but especially Judy, began getting pressure to start a family. There were subtle hints that they were becoming too selfish and if they waited much longer, it would be difficult to adjust to the demands of children. Their friends were settling down, moving to the suburbs, and having babies. They were beginning to feel like social outcasts. What Steve and Judy experienced were the subtle and not so subtle cultural expectations and pressures to begin a family. Steve was more interested in having children than Judy. She enjoyed her career, their couple freedom, flexible lifestyle, and felt little inclination to become pregnant. They had to defend and justify their choice to themselves, families, and friends. They felt—and rightly so—that this was a legitimate decision. Steve had a vasectomy at thirty-four.

MYTHS IN FAMILY PLANNING

In considering family planning, there is no all-purpose, right decision. Be aware of common myths concerning children:
1. The more the merrier.
2. An only child is usually maladjusted.
3. You must have your first child by thirty.
4. Under no circumstances should you have children after forty.
5. It is crucial to have both boys and girls.
6. Planning children takes the love and spontaneity out of sex.
7. Having children stabilizes a rocky marriage.

We suggest the following guidelines for family planning:
1. Having children is a choice agreed to by both spouses.
2. The marriage is on a solid foundation emotionally, sexually, and financially before having a child.
3. Wait at least two years before beginning a family.
4. Children are planned and wanted.
5. Children are at least an eighteen-year commitment. The couple should consider their financial resources and psychological willingness to make this commitment.

CONTRACEPTION AND STERILIZATION

There is no perfect contraceptive. A perfect contraceptive would have the following characteristics: (1) be totally effective, (2) have no immediate or long-term side effects, (3) be separate from sexual activity, (4) easily reversible, (5) require little effort on the part of the user, (6) could be used by male or female, (7) be inexpensive. Nothing presently available comes close to meeting these criteria.

There are two categories of contraceptives, hormonal and barrier. The major hormonal methods are birth control pills, Depo-Provera injections, and Norplant. The major barrier methods are the condom, diaphragm, cervical cap, I.U.D., and vaginal spermicides.

The birth control pill—the most popular contraceptive—is the most effective. The pill must be taken daily and functions by preventing ovulation. Lower levels of estrogen have made the pill safer, with reduced side effects. It is important to choose a gynecologist who is knowledgeable about current research and different brands of pills. It is crucial for the gynecologist to know your full medical history and to monitor your health on a yearly basis. Women who have a family history of blood clotting or stroke are not good candidates for the pill, nor are women over thirty who smoke. For the majority, the birth control pill is a safe and effective means of contraception. A major advantage is that the pill separates the contraceptive act from the sexual act. The woman has to be motivated to take the pill each day. If one is forgotten or missed, take it as soon as possible. If more than twenty-four hours have elapsed, utilize a back-up contraceptive for the rest of the cycle.

Depo-Provera injections (given every three months) are preferred by women who find taking a daily pill difficult. Although convenient, many women find side effects, especially nausea and breakthrough bleeding, hard to adapt to.

Norplant implants have the major benefit of contraceptive protection for up to five years after the gynecologist inserts them. Although cheaper in the long run, it is a major financial expense upfront as well as a commitment to not having children for at least five years. Some women find the side effects, especially weight gain and altered menstrual periods, hard to adjust to.

There is a major concern about the difficulty of removing the implants.

The diaphragm is one of the oldest forms of birth control. It has two major advantages: it is effective when used properly and has virtually no side effects. A gynecologist must properly fit the diaphragm, which is a dome-shaped thin rubber cup stretched over a flexible ring. The diaphragm blocks conception in two ways. It serves as a barrier covering the cervix so sperm cannot penetrate. Just as vital, a spermicidal jelly is placed around and inside the diaphragm which serves to kill sperm. The spermicide needs to be placed on the diaphragm and the diaphragm inserted into the vagina no sooner than two hours, and preferably closer to an hour, before beginning intercourse. It must be left in place at least six hours after ejaculation. If you desire to have intercourse a second time, you must use a special inserter to apply another dose of spermicide while the diaphragm remains in place. The key to optimal use is the commitment to use it on every occasion no matter how aroused you are.

Condoms are experiencing revived popularity because they are the only contraceptive that protects against STDs and HIV/AIDS. Condoms are the only male contraceptive. Couples who value shared responsibility employ the condom in conjunction with the diaphragm, foam, or spermicides. Some couples begin intercourse and, as arousal builds, withdraw and put on a condom. This is unsafe. Proper use of condoms includes putting the condom on before insertion, leaving a small space at the end to catch the ejaculate, and being sure the male withdraws immediately after ejaculation and holds the condom at the base of the penis so it doesn't spill or slip off. Although condoms are safe, readily accessible, and good contraceptives, they are not as effective as the pill, Depo-Provera, Norplant, diaphragm, or IUD. The female condom has recently been introduced for use with single women, but is not as easy or effective as the male condom.

The IUD is one of the most controversial contraceptives because one type, the Dalkon Shield, was defective, resulting in serious injury to many women. Newer and safer IUD models have been introduced, but the IUD has not regained its popularity. It is crucial to consult a gynecologist who is current on IUD research and skilled at insertion. It is not clear precisely how the

IUD works, but it interferes with the implantation of the ovum in the uterus. Those who are successful with the IUD feel they have effective contraception without worrying about taking a pill each day or inserting a diaphragm before each intercourse. However, because of concerns about its safety and heavy menstrual bleeding it sometimes causes, the IUD is not widely used.

The reason sterilization is the most popular form of birth control for couples over thirty-five is they've become frustrated with and discouraged by contraception. Yet, to avoid an unwanted pregnancy, the answer is a couple commitment to regular use of contraception. Approximately forty percent of marital pregnancies are unplanned, although that does not mean the baby is unwanted. Twenty percent of abortions are performed on married women.

The decision to undergo sterilization should not be made lightly. Although microsurgery has made it easier to reverse a vasectomy, vasectomy and tubal ligation are best thought of as permanent methods. Whether a man should get a vasectomy or a woman have a tubal ligation is a difficult, complex decision. If the couple are sure they do not want additional children, they discuss carefully the range of factors—medical, psychological, sexual, and motivational—to determine who should undertake surgery. The spouse who is more committed to not having additional children, less vulnerable to psychological or sexual worries, and more confident about surgery, is the one who should volunteer. From a medical viewpoint, the vasectomy is the simpler, safer, and less costly procedure. Paradoxically, three times more women have tubal ligations than males choose vasectomies. This is a side effect of the double standard in which conception, contraception, and children are viewed as the responsibility of women.

ENJOYING PREGNANCY AS A COUPLE

It takes two to conceive a child, so there is every reason to join together during the pregnancy: in prepared-childbirth classes, in the delivery room, and in parenting the baby. The traditional view is that childbirth and babies are strictly the concern of women, with men having minimal involvement. It is no wonder the most common time for a couple to separate or for a man to begin an extramarital affair is three months before or three months after the birth of a first child. He feels left out of the pregnancy, her life, and has no sexual outlet. Let us look at a couple where problems were discussed and dealt with in a healthy manner.

Jack and Roberta

In the heat of passion, Jack and Roberta had forgotten to use a diaphragm, and she became pregnant. After a great deal of discussion, they decided that, although the pregnancy was not planned, they did want this child. Roberta had a strong desire—and with some prodding, Jack agreed—for both of them to be actively involved in the childbirth process. They chose an obstetrician and hospital who were enthusiastic about prepared-childbirth and encouraged the husband to be present in the labor and delivery room. They enjoyed taking the childbirth course, practicing exercises at home, and discussing the transitions a new baby would bring to their lives.

Roberta and Jack communicated sexual feelings and needs. Like many couples, they found that Roberta was sexually responsive during the second trimester (due to an increase in pelvic vasocongestion as well as relief over no longer having morning sickness). Roberta was thrilled to be multiorgasmic for the first time in her life.

As Roberta became larger and felt awkward during the last trimester, they discussed alternative intercourse positions and nonintercourse sexual expression. Their favorite late-stage intercourse position was Roberta sitting on the sofa with a pillow supporting her back with her vulva at the edge of the sofa. Jack knelt on three cushions, both for comfort and so his penis was directly in front of her vagina. There was no pressure on Roberta's stomach, a crucial factor during late pregnancy. Jack could fondle her breasts, mons, and clitoral area. Roberta could massage Jack's testicles and inner thighs during coitus. They liked the sitting-kneeling position so well they continued using it after the pregnancy. They also used side by side intercourse positions and especially liked the side rear entry position where there was minimal pressure on her uterus.

There were times Jack wanted to be sexual, but Roberta felt

uncomfortable or wasn't interested. Those times, she would manually or orally stimulate him to orgasm. Other times, he would masturbate while she held him. Roberta made it clear that even when she felt heavy, awkward, and not sexual, she still desired affectionate touching. She liked being stroked and held, and took pleasure from satisfying Jack. Roberta and Jack valued the closeness they shared during pregnancy.

The birth of their daughter was one of the peak experiences in Jack and Roberta's lives. Although it was not pain-free, the classes and exercises paid off. Roberta experienced a great deal of fulfillment in being awake and alert at the birth. Jack's involvement was more gratifying than he'd anticipated. Being Roberta's coach and supporter was much more fulfilling than the role of an inept father pacing in the waiting room. Roberta remained in the hospital two days, and they had "rooming in." This allowed them to become accustomed to the tasks of parenthood—changing diapers, breast feeding, and gaining confidence being with the baby.

In the transition to being a family, don't lose track of the husband-wife bond, including your sexual relationship. Motherhood does not mean the woman becomes asexual. Couples need to devote time to reestablishing sexuality while being cognizant of the stresses and strains of parenting. Three of four couples report decreased sexual frequency and vitality, but this doesn't have to be a self-fulfilling prophecy. The year after childbirth is a hard time for couples; it certainly was for us (our first child was a nonsleeper). Sleep deprivation inhibits sexual desire. Talk about how to cope with this transition so you look back on the experience as one which strengthened your bond rather than subverted it.

Having children is a choice. We predict that in the future more couples will choose not to have children. Not having the responsibility of parenting allows greater degrees of freedom in a couple's lifestyle, career plans, financial status, and ability to travel. Children are a great financial as well as emotional responsibility, especially if viewed as a burden instead of a choice. The primary reason to have children is a genuine desire and commitment to the growth and development of another human being. Having children is a commitment to share yourselves emotionally, physically, financially, and psychologically for at least eighteen years.

INFERTILITY

Approximately twenty percent of couples have difficulty conceiving. Infertility problems put inordinate stress on the marital bond, partly because they are so unexpected. Couples assume they will have no trouble becoming pregnant. It is extremely upsetting and frustrating to discover that what is so easy for so many people is difficult and could prove impossible for you. If you are one of the one in five couples facing infertility problems, the first guideline is not to blame yourself or question your masculinity/femininity.

There are a host of causes for fertility problems. Those that affect women include failure to ovulate, blocked fallopian tubes, an incompetent cervix, vaginal acidity, endometriosis, and vaginismus. About forty percent of fertility problems involve male disorders, which include low sperm count, erectile dysfunction, poor sperm motility, and ejaculatory inhibition. A fertility problem is best viewed as a couple problem, not a cause for blame or guilt. Infertility puts enormous stress on the person's sense of well-being, the couple bond, and sexual relationship. If you have not conceived after twelve months of trying, we suggest an evaluation with an infertility specialist. If the problem is not resolved in nine months, we suggest consulting a marital therapist and/or an infertility support group to help you deal with the psychological, relational, and sexual stress caused by fertility problems.

A specific problem is isolated and easily treated for one in four couples. The remainder have to deal with medical assessment and intervention techniques, including drugs to promote ovulation, microsurgery to open fallopian tubes, varicocele surgery or hormone treatment to improve sperm functioning. Couples engage in sex therapy to deal with inhibited sexual desire, vaginismus, erectile dysfunction, or ejaculatory inhibition. Artificial insemination with either the husband's or a donor's sperm is successful for many couples. There are a number of expensive and difficult technological alternatives, such as *in vitro* fertilization. Unless one has experienced this, it's hard to imagine the individual and couple stress caused by a fertility problem.

Margaret and Frank

Margaret had an unplanned pregnancy at sixteen. After talking with her parents and consulting the minister, Margaret decided to continue the pregnancy and give the baby up for adoption. Although this was an emotionally painful experience, she hoped to become pregnant and have a planned, wanted child after she was married. She was proud to have graduated high school with her class and expected to marry after completing college.

Margaret entered her twenties as Americans were undergoing a dramatic change in patterns of dating and marriage. She married Frank (who was thirty-two, this was his second marriage) when she was twenty-eight. Frank wanted to wait at least three years before beginning a family. When they began having intercourse without contraception, Margaret was enthusiastic and optimistic. Her enthusiasm turned to frustration and then panic when they did not become pregnant. Margaret was thirty-three and terrified she would not be able to have children.

The infertility specialist they consulted was technically expert, but not empathic or forthcoming (a typical complaint about infertility specialists). Margaret and Frank chose to stay with him because of his excellent professional reputation, but decided to consult a marital therapist to deal with emotional stress, discuss alternatives, and resolve conflicts. Medical assessment indicated that Frank's sperm were impaired in terms of motility, there was blockage in Margaret's fallopian tubes, and the post-coital test indicated Frank's sperm were not progressing through the cervix in sufficient numbers. As the months rolled by, Frank felt sexual pressure, which resulted in erectile dysfunction during the high probability week. Intercourse on a timetable lowered Margaret's sexual desire. The marriage therapist suggested that Margaret and Frank emphasize pleasurable, spontaneous sex during the rest of the month. They needed that time to reenergize intimacy and their sexual bond. This was helpful, the task-oriented sex of the high-probability week was no fun.

The marital therapist suggested trying insemination with Frank's sperm. The infertility specialist reinforced this strategy.

Insemination is a more successful way of becoming pregnant than intercourse. Frank and Margaret were ambivalent—Frank because he saw it as a sign of failure, and Margaret because it seemed clinical. However, as they discussed feelings and perceptions, they became comfortable with the idea. They scheduled two inseminations during the high probability week, and were encouraged to have intercourse after the second insemination. They were not sure whether the resulting pregnancy came from insemination or intercourse, and they didn't care.

Anita and Jonathan

Jonathan was an accountant, a very precise fellow. He didn't like leaving things to chance, so when they decided to get pregnant he insisted they employ fertility enhancement procedures. They used an over-the-counter device to determine when Anita ovulated. They had intercourse three days before she was to ovulate, the day before, and the day of ovulation. Jonathan had read it was important to have intercourse in the man-on-top position, that he thrust deeply and withdraw immediately after he ejaculated, and she stay in that position with her knees bent for twenty minutes to facilitate the sperm swimming through the cervix. They followed this format rigorously for six months. When she did not become pregnant, Jonathan insisted they consult an infertility specialist. He willingly gave a sperm sample with the full expectation that it would be fine. Jonathan was anxious to go ahead with testing of Anita to pinpoint the problem, but was shocked to discover he produced very few sperm. The prognosis for him to cause conception was negative. He consulted two urologists with a subspecialty in infertility who confirmed this. Jonathan was used to feeling in control of his life, his profession, and ability to make numbers come out right. He was dismayed he couldn't do this in an area that seemed as easy and natural as conception.

Anita's emotional strength helped them through this crisis. Anita valued Jonathan as a spouse, lover, and person. There is no connection between fertility and masculinity or sexual prowess. Anita valued their sex life, but had found the pregnancy enhancement procedures off-putting. She initiated sexual play more during the month following the sperm count than at any other time in the marriage. Jonathan was hesitant, but as Anita emphasized the importance and quality of their sexual relationship, Jonathan emerged from his depression and became a fully involved intimate partner.

Anita took the lead in discussing alternative means of becoming a parent. They considered adopting a hard-to-place older child, using insemination with donor sperm, adopting a foreign infant, trying surrogate parenting, and having foster children. Although these alternatives work for other couples, Jonathan and Anita opted to proceed with adoption. Jonathan joked that between writing an autobiography, going through a detailed personal and family history, having a social worker visit and assess their home, and getting letters of reference, adopting a child was a much more rigorous procedure than biologically having a baby. The adoption process certainly causes the couple to carefully consider their motivation to parent. If couples had to do this before becoming pregnant, many would opt to remain childless. Anita and Jonathan maintained their motivation and "jumped through the hoops." The process took over two years—they adopted a six-month-old girl and two years later a one-month-old boy.

CLOSING THOUGHTS

Conception, contraception, and infertility are among the most complex and value-laden issues a couple faces. Discussing attitudes, values, feelings, and reaching a decision both people can live with is vital. One of the most important decisions a couple makes is whether to have children, and, if yes, when and how many. The process involves values, attitudes, and, most important, the emotional commitment of both people. We are strong advocates of planned, wanted children. Although that's the ideal, unfortunately it's the exception rather than the rule.

No matter what decision you make, remember you are a couple first. The most important relationship in a family is the husband-wife bond. If you keep it strong and satisfying, parenting will go better for you as well as the children.

9

PARENTS AS SEX EDUCATORS

Children are sexual from the day they're born. Within a few hours, even minutes, of birth females vaginally lubricate and males have an erection. Children are aware of their bodies and genitals at a very young age. Sexual feelings exist throughout childhood and greatly increase during adolescence. Parents who deny sexual realities face a crisis as the children become adolescents and young adults.

The sexual issues and conflicts adolescents experience exacerbate the concerns of parents. Behind most parents' concern is *fear*—fear the adolescent will contract HIV/AIDS, become pregnant, be sexually abused, or be emotionally damaged in a destructive relationship. Parents hope to delay the onset of sexual problems by ignoring their children's sexuality, a useless and self-defeating strategy. Parents who do not have a good sexual relationship or had harmful sexual experiences in childhood or adolescence find this aspect of child development conflictual, bringing forth feelings of personal and parental inadequacy.

To eliminate the cycle of fear and conflict, the first priority is for parents to develop an understanding of, and comfort with, their own sexuality. Parents who provide a positive model of knowledge and comfort establish an excellent base for family sex education. Perhaps the best sex education for a child is to see Mom and Dad kissing in the kitchen or being affectionate in the family room. Parents who verbally and behaviorally give a clear, positive message about touching provide a solid basis for the child's view of relationships and sexuality. Parents who are aware they are not only mother and father, but also husband and wife, are better able to deal with family sexuality issues.

Marge and John

Marge and John had been married twenty-seven years. For the past eight they'd had sexual difficulties because of John's intermittent erectile dysfunction. During the last two years John had been unable to have intercourse, which finally caused them to consult a sex therapist. Partly because of parental discomfort, the children's sex education was "education by omission." There were few sex talks between mother and daughter or father and son. Parental sex education consisted of vague warnings to "stay out of trouble." Marge and John regretted being neither positive sex educators nor askable parents. At the time of treatment, their son was twenty-five and the daughter twenty-one, both unmarried.

Sex therapy was successful because John and Marge cared about each other and were open to learning new communication and sexual techniques. Like many couples with sexual difficulties, the combination of performance anxiety and misunderstanding resulted in a self-perpetuating cycle of anticipatory anxiety, tense and unsuccessful sexual experiences, and sexual avoidance. The outcome was a decrease in communication and affection. They replaced this self-defeating pattern with openness, intimate communication, nondemand touching, pleasure orientation, and erotic stimulation. John and Marge regained comfort and confidence with erections, allowing sex once again to be a satisfying part of their marital bond. It is not loss of physical ability to function, but loss of comfort and confidence that causes erectile problems.

This newfound comfort extended to telling their young adult children that they were seeing a therapist to improve their marital and sexual relationship. Sharing this information had a number of positive effects. The adult children shared their concerns about relationships and fears that Marge and John were disappointed because of their premarital sexual activity. John and Marge assured the adult children they were loved and not being judged. They did reaffirm their belief that sex reached its ultimate satisfaction in an intimate, committed marriage.

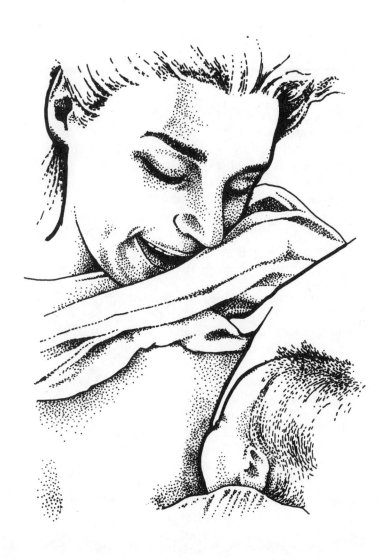

Breast-feeding helps the mother-child bonding process and can be very fulfilling for the woman.

The entire family would have benefited if John and Marge had attended to their sexual relationship earlier. Such attention not only would have helped them as husband and wife, but provided the whole family with an open and comfortable basis for discussing sexual attitudes and values, and being sex educators for their children.

FAMILY SEXUALITY ISSUES

Even when adults are not doing well sexually—they have divorced, the partners are not close, one parent continues to feel victimized by childhood sexual trauma, there has been an extramarital affair, or there is a sexual dysfunction—parents can still provide information, positive attitudes and values to their children. Information has more impact if the parents are a good marital and sexual model. However, parents are people first, who may have difficult relationships or sexual issues in their lives. Being a parent does not mean you pretend to be perfect and have all the answers.

Family sexuality education is a continual process. The child's sex education begins at the moment of birth. Sex is a lifelong, natural physiological function, like breathing. Both parents can touch and hold the baby. The experience of contact comfort allows the child to learn about caring, trust, and security. Feeling good about one's body and enjoyment of touching forms the basis of sexual functioning, and begins early in life. This is equally true for male and female babies. In our culture, male babies receive less holding and cuddling. We encourage father and mother to hold and touch male and female children.

Before the child is a year, she begins exploring her genitals, a natural aspect of body awareness. Since there are more nerve endings in the genitals than other parts of the body, the child experiences pleasure from genital touching. Instead of the parent becoming anxious, slapping the child's hands, and saying "no"—a negative message about her body and touching—the parent accepts body exploration as natural and healthy. The child learns proper words: penis and vulva rather than "dingdong," "down there," or "whatsit." Traditionally, a girl was told she was different from her brother because she lacked a penis. It is better to say, "You are a girl and you have a vulva, your brother is a boy and he has a penis."

As children develop, especially in the four-to-six age range, issues regarding privacy, nudity, and genital touching come to the forefront. The parental message continues to be positive. The child can be comfortable with his body, genitals, and nudity, but learn that there are appropriate and inappropriate contexts and times to express it. Guidelines are individualized, governed by the parents' value system and comfort level.

Judy and Bob

Judy and Bob were raised in homes where nudity was not allowed and displays of affection were restricted to special events, such as birthdays, and consisted simply of a hug and kiss on the cheek. This childhood training had different effects on them due to different sexuality socialization processes for males and females. Bob was a sexually active adolescent who bragged about being a happy warrior in the sexual revolution. He engaged in foreplay not for his enjoyment, but to seduce a woman. When he became erect, he believed he had to have an ejaculation, otherwise the woman was a tease and he was angry at her for playing games.

Judy felt ambivalent about sexuality, although she engaged in premarital intercourse with several partners. She approached sex with anxiety and a desire to please the male, not for her pleasure. She enjoyed kissing, hugging, and caressing because it made her feel cared for and loved. In part, she was compensating for the lack of physical contact in her family. On occasion, especially early in a relationship, Judy was aroused and orgasmic, but did not maintain a sense of comfort, sexual desire, or enjoyment.

Judy and Bob's sexual relationship was exciting premaritally, but became less satisfying during the first year of marriage. Bob had a series of brief extramarital affairs to provide sexual variety and excitement. Judy became involved in a romantic, largely platonic, affair that caused her to consider leaving Bob. She decided against it because they had two young children and she genuinely loved Bob. However, she did not feel loved by him nor sexually attracted to him. His reaction to her affair and the threat of divorce led them to seek marital therapy.

In the course of therapy, it became clear how Bob and Judy's misunderstandings about male-female roles, affection, and sexuality interfered with intimacy. At first, Bob contended he had no sexual problems, but during therapy became aware he had an intimacy problem. He needed to learn to feel comfortable touching, self-disclosing, and being sensual with Judy. Bob had to learn to view sexuality as part of their relationship, not separate from it. Most important, he had to realize that sex and affection were good in themselves, not as ways to demonstrate masculinity or win a woman over. Bob learned to self-disclose, be emotionally vulnerable, and cherish intimate sexuality. Judy had to learn that touching, affection, pleasuring, eroticism, intercourse, and orgasm were a continuation of the same process, rather than viewing affection and sex as two altogether different ways of feeling. Most important, she was to accept sex as pleasing for herself, not just for Bob. She gave herself permission to be a sexual woman, with her own sexual voice.

After eight months of therapy, Bob and Judy developed positive, integrated attitudes about their relationship and marital sexuality. Bob was comfortable being affectionate and sharing intimate feelings, Judy was open to initiating sex and using a variety of erotic scenarios and techniques.

Judy and Bob resolved to provide their children with a positive sex education, better than what they'd received. In this, they are among a large majority of parents. Over eighty percent of couples want to provide their children a healthy sex education. Bob and Judy felt comfortable hugging and kissing not only in the bedroom, but also in the kitchen and living room. In public, they held hands and were affectionate. At first the children were surprised and annoyed at their parents' behavior, especially five-year-old Carol, who said it was "silly" and "gross." Yet both children enjoyed receiving kisses and hugs, especially family hugs.

Although squeamish at first, Judy and Bob accepted their children's growing sexual awareness and questions. When Brent, their six-year-old, was found playing with his penis in front of Carol, they did not panic or fear he would become a sexual deviant. They accepted this as normal childhood sex play, talked to the children about the differences between a penis and vagina, telling them one was not better than the other. They made it clear that running around nude outside, forcing other children to take off their clothes as a prank, and touching genitals in public was not appropriate. They made a clear distinction between sexual play/exploration and sexual coercion/humiliation.

Judy and Bob tried to give their children positive messages about their bodies and genitals. They wanted the guidelines to be appropriate, not permissive. They did *not* engage in sensual or sexual activity in the presence of the children, encourage the children to touch themselves in front of the picture window, or encourage other children to play sex games. These parental behaviors are inappropriate, intruding on the child's autonomy and privacy. Inappropriate parental guidelines cause the child to be hurt and ridiculed by adults and other children. Overly permissive and intrusive handling of sex issues can be just as harmful as overly restrictive and punishing parental behavior.

CHILDHOOD SEXUAL DEVELOPMENT

Contrary to popular mythology, there is *not* a sexual latency period. During the period from six to puberty (puberty begins between 10 and 16) the child is aware of sexuality issues. Children of seven or eight have boyfriends or girlfriends and talk about whom they will marry when they grow up. If a friend's parents divorce, your child will worry that you could divorce too.

The most common time for child sexual abuse is between ages eight and twelve. Parents need to give clear directions to children about their right to say no to an adult who tries to touch their breasts, genitals, or buttocks, or the adult asking or coercing the child to touch him. Most cases of sexual abuse occur not with strangers but with people the child knows. These include neighbors, church personnel, playground aides, relatives, teachers, boy scout leaders, school personnel, or youth group leaders. Sexual abuse occurs with male as well as female children. The child needs to know that if there is an incident or she has questions or concerns, she can come to you and you will believe and help rather than be angry or reproachful.

Intrafamily sexual abuse is a very complex, difficult, emotional topic. Uncles, brothers, stepfathers, in-laws, grandfathers, cousins, and stepbrothers are possible perpetrators of sexual abuse. Father-daughter incest is most traumatic because it is a violation of the trust bond and becomes the ''shameful family secret.'' We encourage fathers to be more involved and affectionate with their children. However, there is a clear line between affectionate touching and sexual abuse. Affectionate touching is nongenital, a sign of caring, and shows respect for the child's person and feelings. Sexual abuse involves genital touching, is done to meet the sexual needs of the perpetrator at the expense of the child's emotional needs, and is secretive.

One in three female children and one in seven male children are sexually abused. Most abuse is not violent, nor does it involve intercourse. Parents need to talk to their child about sexual abuse, and make it clear she can ask questions or reveal an incident. You will listen, help, and protect her.

The preadolescent is becoming increasingly aware of himself and will want privacy when bathing and undressing. At the same time, he is becoming more aware of parents' sexual activity. The child is torn between natural curiosity and embarrassment. Giving both parents and children privacy is the preferred way to deal with this. At the same time, you want to be an approachable, affectionate parent. The most important guideline is to be an ''askable parent.'' Be willing to discuss issues and questions on the child's level of comprehension.

Harold and Susan

Harold and Susan's children were eleven, nine, and six. A house rule was that mom and dad had private time. Unless there was something urgent, they were not to be disturbed. One component of private time were talks over a cup of coffee at the kitchen table after dinner. While they were talking, the children did homework, music practice, or played. If the phone rang one of the older children answered and took a message.

Another component of private time involved Harold and Susan's bedroom. When the door was open, the children knew they could come in and usually did. However, when the door was closed, the children went about their business, took phone messages, and did not interrupt. When the kids were younger, Harold and Susan put a lock on their bedroom door, and they continue to use it (a lock on the parents' door is highly recommended).

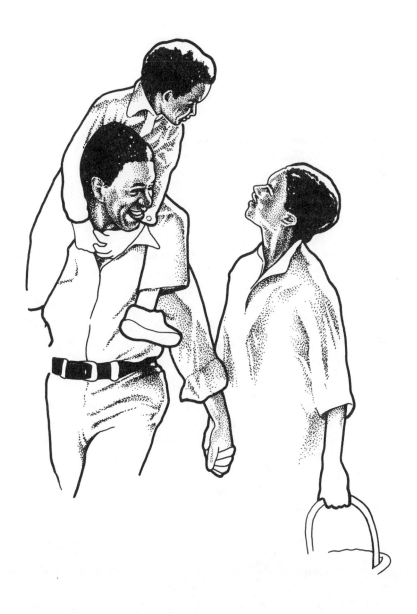

Being affectionate in front of your children and with your children is an important sex education message.

At times, they would go to their bedroom to read. Sometimes they would have intercourse, and other times relax, talk, give a back rub, or engage in pleasuring. Although most of their sexual activity occurred when the children were asleep, they particularly enjoyed sexual experiences when they had time and energy. In response to the children's curiosity, Harold and Susan said, "We need time together. We love you and enjoy being your mother and father. We love each other and enjoy being married. Sometimes when we are in the bedroom we talk, sometimes we share our love, and sometimes we just want time to ourselves."

Harold and Susan were affectionate with each other and the children. There was no sensual or sexual touching or innuendo in front of the children. The eleven-year-old daughter was at an excellent age for sexuality education, but the school program was weak. Susan and Harold took a proactive approach to family sex education. They got books and pamphlets from the library, read them before giving them to their daughter and discussed specific attitudes and behavior. Once the daughter and parents got over initial discomfort, discussing sexual issues from menstruation to contraception to personal values proved worthwhile. Harold and Susan felt better prepared to handle sexuality discussions with the younger children.

FAMILY SEXUALITY EDUCATION

Talking about sex and privacy is one way for parents to give children informal sex education. The child is encouraged to partake of different educational experiences, some formal and some informal. Formal content-based sex education programs offered by schools, value-oriented sex education programs offered by the church or temple, and the informal sex education of talking with peers, are all important. Of crucial importance is family sexuality education.

Sexuality is an important, integral, complex part of a person's life and must be understood with respect for that complexity. The old method of sex education included one film in sixth grade, a litany of "don'ts" from the church, a lot of joking, bragging, and myths passed on by the peer group, and a single father-son or mother-daughter talk which emphasized not getting "in trouble." This is not the kind of sex education we have in mind, although it is typical of that received by the majority of parents and to a lesser extent their children. Ideally, schools would integrate sex education into the curriculum throughout elementary and high school. Churches would give equal weight to positive values regarding sexuality as well as to sanctions for behavior they judge immoral. Peer groups would be honest and straightforward in discussing sexuality, including admitting uncertainties and confusion, sharing information and experiences, rather than bragging and forcing experimentation in order to "be cool." We have a long way to go before we reach this level of sex education.

Family sexuality education is not a one-shot lecture. It is a continuing process of sharing information, exploring feelings and perceptions, and discussing value-oriented issues. In addition to father-son and mother-daughter talks, it includes each parent talking to the child as well as family discussions with both male and female children. More than the mechanics of sexuality—physiology, disease, and conception—need to be covered. Discussions include feelings, values, and attitudes about a range of topics from masturbation to intercourse, from contraception to STDs and HIV/AIDS

There is a tendency to emphasize risks and harm because this is what parents fear. Sexual abuse, STDs, HIV/AIDS, sexual assault, and unwanted pregnancies are crucial issues to deal with, but the initial and primary focus should be on the positives of touch and sexuality, not the negatives. You don't want your children to be afraid of sex. You want them to be aware, knowledgeable, and comfortable. As in other areas of life, knowledge is power. A knowledgeable child is likely to be sexually responsible.

Be sure to orient information to the level of the child's interest and understanding. As in other areas, such as how to handle money or how a car works, you deal with increasing levels of complexity as the child develops. When a seven-year-old asks what inflation means, it is confusing and inappropriate to review Keynesian versus laissez-faire economic theories. Explain sexual issues to her as clearly as possible. Talk to a seven-year-old on his level. When he asks why he gets a "boner", don't commence describing the relationship between mental images and vasocongestion.

Parents say they are ready to answer any question, but the child doesn't ask. It is your responsibility to be an "askable parent." Raise issues and discuss the child's sexual and relationship concerns. Convey information and perceptions without being intrusive or forcing the child to reveal private matters. The child needs to feel she can share information or ask questions, and you will listen and respond. Sometimes children want to have an involved, serious conversation; other times they'll share a joke or observation. Listen to their needs.

The ideal parental message is that sexuality is a positive part of life, integral to being a female or male, and that sexuality enhances the person's life. Discuss sexual experiences that can harm their lives, such as an unwanted pregnancy, being sexually victimized or harassed, rejected in a relationship, feeling inadequate, a negative body image, guilt over masturbation or fantasies, not being comfortable as a male or female. Parents state as clearly as possible their views regarding masturbation, dating, sexual touching, premarital intercourse and contraception. The adolescent does not have to—and well may not—share the parents' values, but at least he is aware of them. Discuss values regarding marriage, family planning, and—if you feel comfortable—marital sexuality.

Empirical research indicates years thirteen to sixteen are the most unhappy time in a person's life. The second most unhappy time is between nineteen and twenty-two. A good portion of the conflict revolves around life decisions, including sexuality. These are periods of experimentation, transitions, and increased independence. Adolescents and young adults are attempting to develop their own identities and lives. Not surprisingly, one of the most stressful periods for a couple is when their children are adolescents. Transition periods are difficult for all concerned. You can best handle these by communicating, stating feelings and limits, and maintaining your role as an approachable parent—someone to turn to if there's trouble, with a question, or to share feelings.

Julia and Mike

Julia and Mike have two children, sixteen-year-old Karen and fourteen-year-old Rob. When the children were younger, nudity was accepted in the home. Julia and Mike were affectionate with each other and the kids. Books and pamphlets about where babies came from, the development of the human body, sexual abuse prevention, and differences between males and females were readily available.

When Karen began dating at fifteen, there were discussions about how late she would stay out, where she could go, and whom she dated. Julia and Mike wanted to do more than set rules. Julia told Karen she could and should enjoy boys, including kissing and touching. Julia shared her strong feelings that going steady or becoming involved in petting to orgasm was not appropriate at this age. She told Karen virginity was not the most important thing in the world, but being good to herself, not getting hurt in a relationship, safeguarding her sexual health, and avoiding pregnancy were crucial. Mike told Karen he was proud she was becoming a young woman and he very much loved her. He tried to give her positive messages about males, for, after all, he was once a young man and her younger brother was someone she cared for. He was frank in saying that many boys use girls to ''score'' and brag of sexual conquests as a way of proving masculinity. Mike told her that no matter what, her parents loved her and she could feel free to come to either one with questions or problems.

In addition to individual talks with Karen, Mike and Julia had family discussions that involved Rob. Sexual values, relationships, AIDS, planning children, and marriage were topics. Julia and Mike strongly believed it was best to delay marriage until young adulthood—twenty-three at the earliest. They wanted the children to have respect for themselves and not hurt or manipulate others for sexual gain. They tried to give Karen and Rob the same guidelines because they believed in a single standard, not the traditional double standard, for sexuality and relationships. They were honest and practical in making them aware of ''sex lines and dating games.'' The children discussed with each other (siblings are important sex educators in the family) their feelings about the double standard and relationships.

To supplement informal discussions, sexuality books were available at the house. These were read and discussed by children and adults. For example, a book or pamphlet could serve as the basis for a discussion about contraception. Mike and Julia mentioned those they had used during marriage, discussing their experiences and weighing positive and negative aspects of each. They encouraged the children to read the chapter on choosing a mate and when to marry. They shared with Karen and Rob their feelings about dating and marriage. Mike talked about his first marriage. He had married at nineteen, had one child, and was divorced by twenty-two. The children were very interested, and Mike discussed what he felt comfortable sharing and chose not to share other things—specifically, that his first wife was six months pregnant when they married.

This points up one of the most difficult dilemmas of the family sexuality approach. The model works best when parents have a good relationship, do not feel guilty about their sexual past, and are comfortable sharing personal experiences. Parents who are disappointed or frustrated with the state of their marriage, have had or are having difficult times in their sexual life, are plagued by feelings of guilt or embarrassment about past behavior, or choose to guard ''family secrets,'' need to ensure these do not dominate the sexuality education of the children.

In deciding what you want to share, recognize and accept your individuality and moral and religious values. There is not one right way to educate children sexually. Consider the views presented as guidelines. Develop a sex education approach based on your history, relationship, comfort, and values. Be aware that ninety-five percent of people have had at least one sexual experience that was confusing, guilt-inducing, or traumatic, and the majority have had several. Feeling embarrassed or guilty about the past is self-defeating. Guilt lowers self-esteem and makes it more difficult to deal with the sex education of your children. Each couple needs to decide what of their past behavior, feelings, and attitudes to reveal. Parents should *not* ''dump secrets'' on children, talk about past sexual escapades, disclose sexual problems, or comment on what arouses them.

It is beneficial for children to realize parents are individual people. This is especially true of divorced, remarried, or single parents. It is healthy for the child to realize that the adult world has its changes, stresses, and transitions. Growing up with the myth that, once you are married, life remains static and ''happy ever after'' is not in the child's best interest.

ONGOING SEX EDUCATION

Sex education is an ongoing process that does not end when children reach eighteen. Both you and they continue to develop and change. Children become independent adults who have lives of their own and are responsible for their decisions. Parents feel overly responsible for adult children's marital and sexual adjustment. A parent has a responsibility to give care and attention to the child, but after age eighteen the person is responsible for his behavior. The parent can provide guidance and serve as a resource but should *not* assume responsibility. The best stance is that of a consultant. Parents should not judge the success of their lives by the accomplishments or problems of their children, whether in sexual, vocational, or marital areas.

The aging parent can serve as a model to the adult child that life does not end at sixty. Affection and sexuality can be enjoyed in the sixties, seventies, eighties, and longer. This is one of the best sex education messages you can give.

10
BEING A COUPLE AGAIN

Children are a major commitment. You are responsible for children for the first eighteen years of their lives. After they leave home, good parents remain vitally interested in and concerned about young adult children.

Raising a child is one of the most rewarding experiences in life as well as one of the most stressful. Parenting requires immense amounts of time, psychological and physical energy, and commitment. Children need consistent, involved, concerned parents. A common trap is to be so involved in parenting that you think of yourselves as parents, not individuals or a married couple. In an extreme manifestation, you call each other ''Mom'' and ''Dad.''

It is crucial to be aware that you are a person in your own right as well as part of an intimate couple. This attitude, if adopted early in the marriage, sets the stage for a positive transition to being a couple again after the children leave home. We wrote this edition when all of our children were young adults, although we are actively involved in grandparenting our four-year-old grandson.

When our children were young, we found parenting very satisfying. We especially enjoyed family outings and vacations. We set a priority on having two weekends a year to go away as a couple without children. This was important when the children were young, but even more so when they were adolescents. We especially remember a week's couple vacation (the children stayed with another family who had children of similar ages, and we reciprocated a month later). During that week we had time to swim, sightsee, make love, sit on the beach, watch sunsets, and plan the first book we wrote together. These experiences kept our marital bond vital as well as prepared us for the transition to being a couple again.

When children become young adults and leave home, whether for college, jobs, the military, or training programs, parents experience the "empty nest" syndrome. This was believed to be a traumatic or at least difficult period of adjustment, especially for women. Recent research and newer conceptualizations challenge this conventional wisdom. Being a couple again is a time of individual growth and increased intimacy. Couples report heightened marital satisfaction and renewed sexual interest. The empty nest phase is a time of transition, but can be enhancing personally and maritally rather than something to dread.

The norm in our culture is to marry in the mid-twenties and have children within three years. Young adult children usually leave home between the ages of eighteen and twenty-three. Most people become a couple again in their late forties or mid-fifties. Of course, there are wide differences: people may enter this life stage in their late thirties and others not until their late sixties. Adult children may return home, sometimes with a grandchild, so the nest becomes cluttered rather than empty.

Couples will have as much, or more, time together as they spent parenting. Be aware, while still in the parental role, of the prime importance of the marital bond. You are first individual, then a married couple, and then parents. People who value individuality and their couple bond are more satisfied with their lives and better parents. Do not make being a couple subservient to being a parent, even when children are young. The most important relationship in a family is the husband-wife bond. If that bond is healthy and satisfying, it makes parenting easier and is in the best interest of the children.

Being a couple again is a crucial transition for your marital and sexual relationship. Like other transitions, it can be a time of increased growth and satisfaction, yet presents potential traps and risks. The more aware you are of opportunities and problems, the better your decision-making and ability to adopt coping strategies. Being a couple again is a time to revitalize your intimate bond.

Alice and Tom

Alice and Tom, a couple in their late forties, very much enjoyed raising their three children. Ralph was twenty-six, married, and involved in his career. Andi was a senior in college, and Jim had just moved out of the house and begun a training program in forestry management. For the first time in twenty-six years there were no children at home, although they visited on weekends and over holidays. The adjustment was more difficult for Alice than Tom, since she had been more involved on a day-to-day basis. Eight years before, she had begun preparing herself for this transition by returning to school and completing an advanced degree in computer programming. She recently received a promotion to systems engineer.

Tom and Alice welcomed the independence and maturity of their children. It allowed them time and freedom to pursue their interests. Alice was invested in her career, she was elected an officer in her professional organization. Tom had greater opportunity to pursue hobbies. With the financial burden lessened and two substantial incomes, they were able to indulge themselves. One of their first purchases was camping equipment for two people instead of a family. They found it freeing to no longer have to schedule weekend trips and vacations around children's school and extracurricular activities. Although Tom and Alice were not emotionally oriented in their couple communication style, they very much enjoyed doing things together and sharing outdoor experiences. Tom bought some long desired photography equipment. Alice enjoyed accompanying him on photography shoots. She was free to travel to seminars on computer management, and had a sense of increased professional competence.

No longer concerned about interruptions from children, their sexual relationship was adventuresome and spontaneous. They discovered that "nooners" were particularly exciting, especially after years of relegating sex to a late-night activity. Lovemaking was creative and flexible. Alice could walk around the house in a bra and panties—or nude, if she desired. Tom experienced a renewed sense of desire as they had sex in the den, necked on the living room couch, made love in the guest bedroom (and slept there through the night).

Alice especially enjoyed prolonged pleasuring. Not having to worry about interruptions from phone calls, children's noise, or knocks on the door ignited sexual desire. Alice would suggest taking a ten-minute break from pleasuring to have a glass of wine. When they returned to erotic stimulation, Alice was receptive and responsive.

Tom enjoyed the opportunity to be sexual in different places, including taking advantage of camping weekends. They went wilderness camping and made love under the stars. Tom relished creative sexual scenarios at home. He enjoyed sexual play in one room and intercourse in a different room. Tom accompanied Alice to her conventions and used these opportunities to compare Hilton and Marriott rooms to see which best promoted a sexually inviting environment.

Alice and Tom continued active interest in parenting. They enjoyed their adult children coming home for Thanksgiving and special occasions. Tom and Alice visited their adult children on their "turf," an implicit acknowledgement that they were independent adults with lives of their own. Alice and Tom talked with them about a variety of matters, including sexual issues. Tom was particularly pleased that Andi and Jim sought his advice about housing and financial decisions. Tom and Alice gave guidance when it was requested, without forcing their views. They recognized Ralph, Andi, and Jim as adults who were responsible for their lives. They loved and were concerned about their adult children, but did not assume the burden of responsibility for their successes and problems. They adopted the role of consultant, not offering advice unless it was requested.

DIFFICULT TRANSITIONS

Not everyone makes a positive adjustment to being a couple again. Problems occur when couple interaction centers chiefly around children. With this topic gone, they have little to talk about. An extreme example is parents who put pressure on adult children to have a baby so they have a grandchild to attend to. They need a child-oriented role as grandparents because they feel awkward and empty being a couple.

Not having anything to communicate and finding few shared interests is a rude awakening. The couple is afraid to admit this is the state of their relationship, because to do so could entail a move toward divorce with its looming loss of the security of more than twenty years of married life. The couple who denies there is a problem cannot put energy into rebuilding the relationship, so it continues to stagnate. Such empty nest marriages are mediocre at best and can disintegrate into lonely, bitter relationships. A sexual dysfunction such as an erection problem, inability to reach orgasm, and/or inhibited sexual desire is likely. Lack of sexual desire leads to general avoidance of affection. The absence of intimacy and touching accelerates alienation.

Couples who admit they have grown apart and are facing serious problems can mobilize their resources and energy toward rebuilding a sharing, communicative marriage. The vitality of a marital bond can and often does dissipate under the stresses of raising teenagers. Confronting this reality allows the couple to begin rebuilding. With the children gone, this is an excellent opportunity to deal with each other and set the stage for being a satisfying couple again in marriage.

Donna and Jeff

Donna and Jeff were a struggling couple who had become so used to practical problems and adolescent hassles that they did not know what to do when they were a couple again. Donna had three children from her first marriage, which ended when the husband died in a car accident. Four years later she married Jeff, who had two children from a first marriage and one from a second. Jeff's children stayed with them on an intermittent basis. Stepfamilies are not, and should not try to be, a replica of the traditional nuclear family. Blended families have their unique stresses as well as unique strengths and learning opportunities.

Donna and Jeff found adolescent crises draining. They fought about child management, finances, practical matters like who was going to clean up after the dog, and general unhappiness with each other. Donna would become depressed, which coincided with Jeff's abusing alcohol. It seemed anticlimactic for the children to be gone and have a relatively stress-free home life. For a time they considered becoming more involved in their adult children's marriages and assuming responsibility for grandchildren, but wisely decided not to. Although they were willing to help on a temporary basis and in a crisis, too much intervention would interfere with the adult children finding their own solutions.

Jeff and Donna were uneasy being with each other. During the previous ten years they'd engaged in relatively few couple activities. Intercourse had decreased to less than once a month. The first step in revitalizing the couple bond was to accept the reality of the situation. Instead of being worried and fearful, they resolved to make a good faith effort to rebuild intimacy and sexuality.

They went on a week's couple vacation, which turned into a second honeymoon. Jeff and Donna enjoyed the trip and, more importantly, used the time to share feelings and reestablish their sexual relationship. On the last day of vacation, Donna sat the two of them down. She wanted a commitment to continue intimacy and keep sexuality on track rather than their falling into old habits and ignoring the relationship except when there was a crisis.

They settled into the routine of jobs, housework, social engagements, contact with children and grandchildren, and neighborhood activities. Donna and Jeff reserved two evenings a week for couple activities. Sometimes they worked together around the house or watched TV. Other times they went to a movie, had a sexual date, or went for a walk. Intercourse frequency was one or two times per week. They did not strive for the perfect marriage described in magazine articles; they wanted a marriage which met their needs. Donna and Jeff were individualists who resented the notion that marriage was supposed to be communicative and loving twenty-four hours a day, seven days a week. What was important was knowing they could depend on each other, enjoy the other's company, cuddle on the couch, and make love.

Are there marriages based on children or security in which it is not possible to resurrect intimate feelings? Some couples lose touch, or perhaps never had a vital relationship, sex was infrequent or nonexistent. The marriage was functional in meeting companionate, financial, and/or practical needs. Although needs for emotional intimacy and sexual fulfillment were not met, these were not a high priority. There are couples who stay married and are satisfied with the marriage even though there is little or no sexual connection. These couples chose to focus on other rewarding aspects of their lives. In fact, one in five married couples have a nonsexual marriage.

GUIDELINES FOR REVITALIZING YOUR INTIMATE BOND

Couples who value intimate sexuality can implement the following guidelines.

1. Acknowledge you are going through a major life transition.
2. Accept your relationship and sexual interests/needs have changed.
3. Sexuality needs to be intimate and interactive, and involve more than intercourse.
4. Commit to put time and psychological energy into the marriage.
5. Be open during sexual play. Sensuality, pleasuring, genital stimulation, and eroticism increase sexual satisfaction.
6. Be aware of yourselves as sexual people and a sexual couple, separate from the parental role.

Revitalizing your relationship requires a genuine commitment to communicate feelings, make clear and direct requests, be open to the spouse's needs and desires, and, most important, live in the present rather than be shackled with disappointments, resentments, and regrets over missed opportunities. One of the worst traps is "if only" thinking. Focus your psychological and sexual energy on the present and future. You can learn from the past, but cannot change it.

For many couples, the major roadblock to revitalizing the sexual bond is their history. You cannot be married to someone for more than twenty years and not have memories of hurt, anger, disappointment, and resentment. The question is whether you allow those to control your life and marriage. In his clinical work, Barry asks each spouse to make a list of incidents that still grate on them. These are relationship "poisons." Then he asks each to state what might be done in the present to alleviate past feelings and change the present situation. The most common request is for the spouse to acknowledge the feelings and offer a genuine apology.

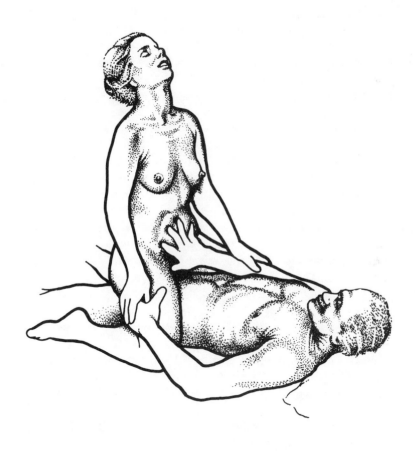

Take advantage of the time and privacy to experiment with prolonged intercourse and multiple stimulation.

ALTERNATIVES TO A REVITALIZED MARITAL BOND

If you find this approach to revitalizing the marital bond is not unacceptable or unproductive, you have several alternatives. One is to decide the marriage does not and will not meet your needs, and consider separation and divorce. A second is to keep the security of the marriage, but develop an independent and autonomous life in which some needs—perhaps including sexual needs—are met outside the marriage. A third alternative is to become involved in the grandparent role and relate to each other as grandparents. The latter role is satisfactory to many couples, although we strongly caution not to put pressure on adult children to produce grandchildren to fulfill your needs. Another alternative is to continue as you have been. There is more to life than emotional intimacy and sexual satisfaction. Friendships, job satisfaction, hobbies, extended family, and social, religious, and community activities provide major gratification. Your marriage continues to meet companionship and security needs.

There is no such thing as a perfect marriage. Each individual and couple has their needs, values, and life situation. You are the only one who can determine what is in your best interest. Your decisions might be somewhat different or, in some cases, entirely different from our guidelines.

Rose and Bill

Rose and Bill have been married thirty-three years. Their youngest child left home to be married at twenty-one. Their three children live in the same neighborhood, and there are six grandchildren. Bill and Rose had an inactive sex life for much of their marriage and have not engaged in intercourse for the past ten years. They are involved in jobs, adult friendships, and church activities. The entire family gathers for Sunday dinner. This ritual is highly valued by Rose and Bill and their extended family. They regularly baby-sit for grandchildren and take one or two grandchildren with them on summer vacation. For Bill and Rose, this is a satisfying marriage and life.

Although they chose a marital style that is contrary to most of the guidelines of this book, it is one that satisfies their needs and is an excellent choice for them. Every couple is unique; there is not one "right" way to attain psychological well-being or marital satisfaction.

Let us consider a couple who attempted to follow our guidelines and found they did not meet their needs.

Nick and Jean

Nick and Jean had two children. When at nineteen their younger daughter went to work in another town, they found themselves, in their late forties and having been married twenty-seven years, feeling awkward about being a couple again. They believed the missing element was communication. They attended a marriage enrichment weekend and read "pop psychology" books. They purchased one of the zanier sex manuals and tried esoteric techniques and positions. Children and friends supported these efforts. Nick and Jean were perceived by friends as a model of a successful couple again.

After eighteen months, they continued to feel dissatisfied with their relationship. After the initial thrill of trying a new technique, they found little pleasure in sex. They were baffled and decided to seek marriage therapy. The clinician tried to help them gain a deeper understanding of themselves and their relationship.

After three months of therapy, the clinician asked them to focus on an issue they had been avoiding for two years—the possibility they had grown so far apart that it really was not possible to revitalize this marriage. Couples badly stretch their marital bond, but it remains intact. However, once a marital bond is broken, i.e., respect, trust, and intimacy are destroyed and they no longer think of themselves as a couple, it is very difficult to resurrect. Nick and Jean had to face a hard choice between holding on to a marriage that would never be more than mediocre or taking a major risk and going their separate ways. It was Jean who decided she wanted more out of life than an unfulfilling marriage. She initiated the separation, and Nick reluctantly agreed. The therapist continued to see Nick to help him work through feelings of disappointment and adjust to being single again. Although the children understood intellectually that their parents would be happier living alone or remarrying, they had great emotional difficulty accepting the decision. That's not unusual; adult children find it difficult to accept parents having lives of their own and undergoing changes, especially marital changes.

CLOSING THOUGHTS

The transition to being a couple again can result in a revitalization of the marital bond and a sense of sexual freedom and spontaneity. Or it can cause personal, marital, and sexual dissatisfaction, with major impact on the couple's life.

Although couples are anxious and unsure about returning to the "couple again" stage, it usually results in increased intimacy and satisfaction. Having opportunities for privacy, increased couple time, and the development of new individual and couple interests is exciting. You can have less inhibited, more creative, spontaneous and intimate sex. Having adolescent or young adult children in the home is confining, inhibiting sensual and sexual expression. It feels delicious, if not illicit, to be in your home with seductive clothing on—or off—and to make love in the den, living room, or even kitchen without fear of children coming home unexpectedly. The couple who learn and grow through this transition have a solid foundation for their aging years. Being a couple again can be satisfying personally, maritally, and sexually. We enjoy this stage of our lives and marriage.

11
SEX AFTER SIXTY

You are a sexual person from the day you're born until the day you die. A couple in good physical health can function sexually into their sixties, seventies, eighties, and longer. How can you reach an understanding of, and positive attitudes toward, the physiological, psychological, marital, and sexual transitions that occur after sixty?

Until recently, the older person consulting a physician or marriage therapist for advice about sexual functioning would be faced with an embarrassed laugh and told either to leave sex to younger people or not to worry since, when sexual functioning wanes, there is nothing to be done. Now, if you consult a well trained professional, you'll find a wealth of information and specific suggestions on making sexuality a positive, integral part of the aging process. Recent research has found that if the couple (1) understand and accept normal changes in sexual functioning that occur with aging, (2) maintain good health and are aware of sexual side effects of medication, and (3) have positive attitudes and are open to a broad-based, flexible approach to sexual expression, their sexual relationship can and will be satisfying.

ATTITUDES TOWARD SEX AND AGING
As with other aspects of human sexuality, the change process involves awareness, acceptance, and communication. The more this occurs through the middle years, the easier it will be to transfer positive attitudes, feelings, and behavior to the later years. Key elements are acceptance of your body image as an

aging person and having an interested and responsive partner. A couple with a history of regular, satisfying sexual expression has a solid basis for continuing pleasurable sex into their older years.

One of the most harmful myths is that males should save their ejaculations because they only have so much semen, and if they overuse it when younger there will be none left. The facts are just the opposite. Men do not run out of ejaculations, nor do women run out of orgasms. The more regular the sexual expression, the easier to maintain sexual functioning. Sex is a natural physiological function and, as with walking, dancing, or playing tennis, the common sense adage is true: "Use it or lose it."

Our culture idolizes youth and beauty. One of the most self-defeating assumptions is that sexual attractiveness depends on a woman being slim and having beautiful breasts and a man being muscular and in athletic shape. If your image of sexuality is based on youthful physical characteristics, you are setting yourself up to feel rejected and sexually unattractive as you age. One's sense of sexual attractiveness is based on enjoying touch, being comfortable with one's body, enjoying the partner and her responsivity, giving and receiving pleasure, and integrating sexuality into one's self-image. Sex is not just intercourse and orgasm, nor does sexuality reside primarily in the genitals. Sexuality is an expression of self-concept, feelings, body image, intimate sharing, and sense of pleasure. Sexuality is integral to who you are as a person and couple. This concept of sexuality is as applicable to the forty- or seventy-year-old as to the twenty-year-old. It forms a healthy basis for lifelong sexuality and facilitates acceptance of a positive body image as you age. Sexuality is subverted by striving to regain youth and beauty. Sexuality belongs to you as a person and is integral to your couple bond.

In Barry's college human sexual behavior course, there is a class on sex and aging with a video showing a couple in their sixties engaging in pleasurable, erotic sexual interactions. After initial discomfort, students find this class a highlight of the course. Realizing an aging couple can enjoy sexuality, continuing to learn and share, is comforting. It removes the pressure to know and experience everything by the time the person reaches twenty-two. The idea that college students have fifty years of sexual experiences to look forward to is liberating. There is sex after college! Viewing sexuality as a lifelong process of giving and receiving pleasure facilitates acceptance of the aging process.

This is certainly a different view of sex and aging than the stereotypic presentation of the "dirty old man" and the "dried up asexual woman." Sex among older people is standard fare for the comedian's repertoire. This perception comes from younger people's anxiety about, and inability to view, older adults as sexual people. In an informal survey taken in the sex class, only one in four students could imagine their parents having sexual intercourse, and only one in twelve could imagine their grandparents being sexually active. Young adults are so used to parents and grandparents telling them not to have sex that it is hard for them to imagine older adults engaging in sex, much less deriving pleasure from it. Adults, whether in their middle years or senior citizens, can improve the image of sex and aging by acknowledging that they are, and enjoy being, sexual.

An extreme example of the denial of sexuality occurs when a parent enters a nursing home. Adult children insist there be no affectionate touching or sexual contact with other residents. The reason for this irrational position is that adult children cannot accept, since they have always denied, the parent's affectional and sexual needs. This is detrimental to those who reside in nursing homes; it denies their right to privacy and the comfort of human contact. The need for human contact is vital from the time you're a baby through the middle years and into your sunset years.

Let us consider a couple who enjoyed their marital and sexual life throughout the middle years and made an easy transition to sexuality and aging.

Pat and Daryl

Pat and Daryl were married when he was twenty-three and she twenty-one. They had three children, the last born when he was twenty-nine and she twenty-seven. This was a typical pattern for their generation.

Pat and Daryl valued their couple bond and throughout the

marriage put energy toward nurturing intimacy and sexual enhancement. At fifty, with their adult children living away from
home, the transition to being a couple again was smooth. They
enjoyed having more time for themselves and each other. Each
valued the spouse's sexual desires and feelings. More than half
their pleasure came from the partner's responsiveness. The "give
to get" pleasure guideline worked well in their marriage. In sexual interactions which were mediocre or unsuccessful—about
one in ten (which is normal for a sexually functional couple)—
they accepted this and laughed about it rather than blaming, being angry, worrying or feeling guilty. Sometimes they had sex
twice in three days, other times they'd go two weeks without
intercourse. Pat and Daryl accepted this variability without worrying about their normality or performance.

As Daryl approached sixty, he needed Pat's direct penile stimulation in order to obtain and maintain an erection. She felt comfortable using a variety of techniques to arouse him, from gently
massaging the shaft to putting his penis in her mouth to stroking
the glans with one hand and massaging his testicles with the
other. They were adept and comfortable with the side-by-side
(scissors) intercourse position as well as the position where her
leg is over his and he enters from the side. From these positions,
Pat found it easier to insert the penis when he was not fully
erect. As intercourse progressed, arousal built, as did the
erection.

They kept a bottle of Aloe Vera handy to use for additional
vaginal lubrication if needed. Daryl became comfortable using
spittle as a lubricant. In their thirties they'd learned that nondemand pleasuring and erotic stimulation were keys to sexual
arousal, knowledge that held them in good stead during the aging
process. Daryl and Pat felt at ease occasionally taking a break
to sip a glass of wine, share feelings, or verbalize sexual fantasies. This pleasurable, nondemand interaction provided a fresh
and varied dimension to their love play and allowed arousal to
build.

Throughout the marriage, Pat had been multiorgasmic during
many of their encounters. As she aged, her orgasmic response
pattern changed. She had been orgasmic five to seven times, and
now experienced one, two, or three orgasms. At times, she would
not be orgasmic. She did not want to force herself or have Daryl

push her to have an orgasm. She respected the rhythm of her sexual needs instead of demanding her body respond as it had when she was forty-five.

Daryl desired to ejaculate only two of the three times they had intercourse. Once or twice he pushed himself to ejaculate even when he did not feel a need, and though he was able to, it was not pleasurable. A week passed before he was receptive to intercourse again. Daryl chose to ejaculate only when he felt the need instead of forcing himself to reach orgasm each time. He explained to Pat that sex was good for him even when he did not ejaculate. Some men feel they achieve a sensation similar to orgasm even though they don't ejaculate. Daryl experienced pleasurable sensations, but was not orgasmic.

Daryl and Pat learned to accept and enjoy sex even when one or both were not orgasmic. Sharing pleasure and intimacy are the prime motives for sex, not orgasm. Orgasm is not always necessary, nor is it the criterion for measuring whether a sexual experience was satisfying.

At times, Pat and Daryl engaged in touching and pleasuring that was sensual but not arousing. This pattern developed early in the marriage when every two months they set aside an evening devoted to nondemand pleasuring which would not end in intercourse or orgasm. This formed the basis for intimate, pleasurable sexuality in their sixties. The strategies and techniques used by Pat and Daryl are well worth considering in your marriage, whether you are thirty, fifty, or seventy. The concepts of intimacy, nondemand pleasuring, and eroticism advocated throughout this book reach their fruition in sex after sixty.

ISSUES IN SEX AND AGING

One of the most harmful myths is that if a couple has any sexual problems, their sex life will necessarily deteriorate and end as they age. For the aware and motivated couple, the opposite occurs. A man who was an early ejaculator can achieve ejaculatory control as part of the aging process. In the older male, ejaculation is a single phase response which facilitates better control.

With a lessened pressure for rapid sexual performance, both men and women can gain greater enjoyment with prolonged sen-

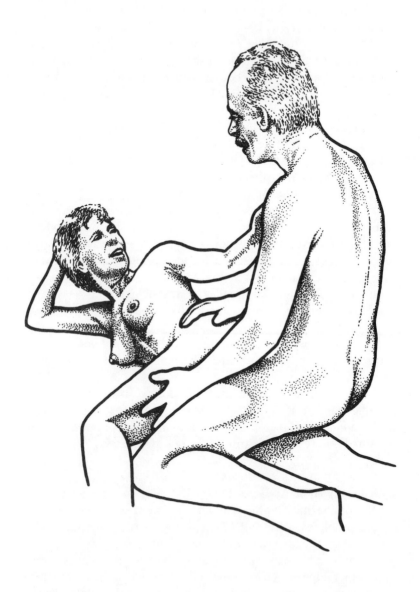

Appreciate a relaxed nondemand approach to touching, sensuality and sexuality. You can be sexual into your sixties, seventies, eighties and beyond.

sual and sexual stimulation. The key elements for effective sexual functioning are nondemand pleasuring, an intimate relationship, the enjoyment of a broad range of erotic scenarios and techniques, understanding and accepting physiological changes, accepting your body image, awareness of altered patterns of sexual response, communicating these to your spouse, engaging in multiple stimulation, and working together to integrate changes into your couple sexual style. This strategy can be adopted by an older couple even if sex in their younger or middle years was dysfunctional.

The most enjoyable clinical case Barry ever saw involved a couple in their sixties who had been married forty-two years. Their marriage had been good in spite of a terribly dysfunctional sexual relationship. They'd read about sex therapy and self-referred themselves to see if anything had changed since their abortive attempt at sex counseling with a physician thirty-eight years ago. They proceeded through sex therapy just like "in the book." The nongenital and genital pleasuring exercises caused an awakening in their bodies. Within two months, she was orgasmic for the first time in her life. Even more than orgasmic response was the pleasure experienced in sharing a passion felt for years but just now expressed.

ILLNESS AND DEATH OF A SPOUSE

Extremely sensitive issues arise when one spouse becomes ill and/or is dying. Death is even more of a taboo subject in our society than sexuality. When you combine the subjects of aging, sex, and death, you have an enormous amount of myth, anxiety and misunderstanding. The more aware and knowledgeable a couple is the easier it will be to deal with these emotionally difficult, complex issues. The best time to think about and discuss these concerns is when both people are healthy, not in the midst of a crisis.

What happens when one spouse becomes extremely, and perhaps terminally, ill? The person's needs for affection and touching continue. To withdraw this contact is to further depress and, in a manner, to abandon the spouse. Contrary to popular myth, affectionate and sensual contact is possible, enjoyable, and enhances the psychological well-being of the ailing person. Even if sexual intercourse is not desired, most ill people, and especially terminally ill people, desire the caring that is expressed through touch.

One factor in adjustment to the spouse's illness involves feelings and attitudes toward masturbation. The majority of married men and women occasionally masturbate. Masturbation is a normal and healthy sexual behavior at any time in life, but especially during a spouse's illness. A harmful myth is that an adult masturbating is indulging in regressive behavior, displaying his senility. Masturbation for a widow or widower is an affirmation of sexuality and a perfectly normal and healthy means of sexual expression.

Couples are well advised to discuss, while still healthy, feelings about dating or remarriage when a spouse dies. This is a value-oriented issue each individual must decide for herself. The spouse does not have to engage in interminable mourning and deny her needs for companionship, affection, and sex. An adage is, "Women mourn while men replace." Both men and women need to mourn, and then consider how to organize their lives. Deciding to be asexual is one alternative open to the survivor. Remarrying, having sex with other partners, masturbating, and being emotionally involved but not sexual with other people are alternatives to consider.

Rita and John

Rita and John were in their late sixties and been married forty-three years when Rita contracted cancer. She underwent surgery, but unfortunately it was too late, the cancer had spread through her body. During Rita's last year of life, they engaged in sexual intercourse, usually at her initiation, about once a month. There were many experiences involving back rubs and lying together. John also used masturbation as a sexual outlet, and although not explicitly discussed, this was accepted by both.

Physical closeness was important as they prepared for her impending death. Two months before she died, intercourse became unpleasant for Rita, but affection and emotional intimacy were desired and continued. Physical closeness facilitated sharing feelings, which included sadness, love, grief, anger, and resignation. This helped Rita better prepare for and accept her death. John was able to express his feelings as well as do the cooking and cleaning to keep the house functional. Holding and talking helped him deal with the grieving process. Engaging in anticipatory grieving while the spouse is alive is emotionally painful, yet psychologically worthwhile, for both people.

When John began a relationship with another woman fourteen months after Rita's death, he had difficulty maintaining an erection. This is to be expected since even though he masturbated he had not attempted intercourse for over a year. As with any physical activity—swimming for example—there is a need to get back into the rhythm of being sexual. This common phenomenon has been labeled the "widower's syndrome." John did not overreact to his temporary erectile problem. He continued to engage in sexual activity that emphasized nondemand pleasuring along with manual and oral stimulation. Instead of avoiding sexual contact, which would have led to performance anxiety and eroded sexual confidence, he continued to engage in pleasure-oriented sexual expression. As his comfort and arousal increased, so did erectile functioning. Eventually, he developed a satisfying sexual relationship, including intercourse, with the new partner. John did not make comparisons between the marriage and this relationship. The best way to approach sexuality and aging, especially in a new relationship, is to be positive. Focus on the new relationship, don't make comparisons with the past.

Juanita and Roy

Juanita and Roy, a couple in their middle forties, had two teenage children. Juanita's parents were alive and married. Roy's mother, a widow, shared her house with a woman friend. Roy and Juanita were committed to keeping their marriage sexually satisfying and raising their children in a sexually healthy environment. They looked forward to being sexual into their sixties and beyond.

Juanita's parents were from the old school, which holds that sex, politics, and religion are three topics never to be discussed. They were not affectionate and had moved to separate bedrooms twenty years before. Not only were they not a good model of an aging couple, Juanita doubted sex had ever been satisfying for her mother. When her father made a comment that Juanita and

Roy would eventually lose their affectionate manner, they were not argumentative but simply said they looked forward to enjoying touching their entire married lives, including when they were grandparents. Their teenage children heard that conversation and understood their parents' message.

Roy's mother had been a widow for over ten years. Roy made it a point to tell her he would accept her dating or remarrying and would not consider this disloyal to the memory of his father. Roy encouraged his mother to do what would make her happy. She did not remarry, although she was active in social groups and had male friends. She confided to Juanita that she felt sexual urges and masturbated to reduce tension, but asked Juanita not to tell Roy. She asked whether Juanita felt an old lady masturbating was perverse. Juanita assured her mother-in-law this was normal and healthy, and shared that she occasionally masturbated—not because she did not love Roy, but to enjoy self-pleasuring as an additional sexual experience. Juanita realized widows have few choices of available men, but urged her to avoid a caretaking relationship with a man.

Roy and Juanita had positive attitudes toward middle-years sexuality and were establishing a base for sexual functioning in the later years. They accepted their aging and the aging of others and were aware that their needs for touching, affection, sensuality, and sexuality would extend throughout their lifetime.

IMAGES OF SEX AND AGING

The negative image of sex and aging is based on the myth that sexual expression of older men is an animalistic, uncontrollable need associated with seeking out younger women or molesting children. These images are exclusively associated with males, as if aging females were sexual neuters. This view of sex and aging is grossly inaccurate. Sexual abuse incidents involve less than two percent of males and primarily involve adolescent and young adult men. More to the point, the need for sexual contact is neither animalistic nor inappropriate, but the result of a natural physiological function and a psychological need for touch and pleasure.

Sexual feelings and expression are normal throughout the life span for both women and men. Touch, affection, sensuality, and sexuality are important in the sixties, seventies, eighties, and beyond. Other sources of pleasure and satisfaction are less available in later years. A person is not as robust physically and no longer has job satisfaction or monetary rewards. Couples have the opportunity to lead a less hectic, less performance-oriented life. They can appreciate a relaxed, nondemand approach to living, including sensuality and sexuality. We need to accept that both touching/affection and eroticism/orgasm are normal and healthy for aging women and men.

The more a couple understands physiological changes in their own and partner's bodies, the better prepared they'll be to adapt their sexual functioning. The most important changes affecting the male are that he no longer has the need to ejaculate at each intercourse, the erection will take longer to develop, he'll need more direct penile stimulation, and the erection will be less firm. After ejaculation, there may be one, two, or more days before he will respond to sexual stimulation. The female typically experiences lessened vaginal lubrication and takes longer to become aroused and reach orgasm.

Physical and sexual changes are gradual rather than dramatic. Contrary to popular myth, changes affect men more than women. There are significant individual differences in the rate at which these changes occur. It is crucial to be aware, accept, and communicate about physiological changes. They do not necessarily lead to a decrease in sexual involvement or satisfaction.

When couples stop having sex, ninety-five percent of the time it is the male who no longer wants to try to be sexual. Couples do not discuss this—it is a non-verbal, unilateral decision. Because of erectile dysfunction, ejaculatory inhibition or inhibited sexual desire, he feels sex is too difficult and not worth it. Traditional male sexual socialization ultimately sabotages his sexual functioning and the couple's sexual relationship. Men and women who are aware and open to viewing sexuality in a broad-based, interactive, pleasure-oriented and intimate team approach continue to have satisfying sensual and sexual experiences throughout their lives.

CLOSING THOUGHTS

As you age, a variety of physical, psychological, relational, and situational changes occur. These changes have both direct and indirect effects on sexual functioning. The more you understand the changes, communicate about and accept them, the easier it will be to maintain a satisfying sexual relationship into your sixties, seventies, eighties, and beyond.

II
DEALING WITH PROBLEMS

12
REVITALIZING SEXUAL DESIRE

At the beginning of a relationship, you feel attracted to and sexually desirous of the new partner. Novelty, illicitness, and romantic ecstasy fill the first few weeks or months of a relationship, an experience not to be missed. However, sexual desire that comes from romantic love seldom lasts two years. It's more likely to disappear after six months. That doesn't mean you've fallen out of love or don't find the partner attractive. What it does mean is that the sexual rush from romantic love is over. Seldom does romantic love/sexual passion last until marriage, much less a year into the marriage.

Intimacy and pleasuring are the enduring sources of marital sexual desire. The immediate stimuli for desire are specific and erotic. They include sexual dreams or fantasies, a sexually-oriented movie or an erotic passage in a novel, an attractive or seductive person on the street, the partner initiating and being turned on, an affectionate or sensual interchange, anticipation of a special sexual encounter. Contrary to popular thinking, long intervals between sex do not build "horniness." A regular rhythm of sexual expression reinforces sexual desire. Like other physical activities—walking, biking, swimming—one has a regular pattern of sexual activity, anticipates, enjoys, and values it. Anticipation, feeling you deserve pleasure, and valuing sexuality is the best way to maintain sexual desire.

The approach we advocate is different from the movie and musical images of romantic love and passionate sex. In the movies there is instant chemical attraction, a tantalizing buildup, and then an explosion of overwhelming, overpowering sexual ecstasy. After seeing an R-rated movie, Barry's clients ask why their sex life can't be like that. Sex is short, intense, nonverbal, with either a new couple or an extramarital affair. The Hollywood scenario sells movies, but makes for disappointing real-life sex. It's a self-defeating model for sexual desire in marriage. The kind of sex that sells in movies is destructive to marital sexuality because it creates unrealistic, unattainable expectations. There are no sexual married couples in the movies.

What are the sources of sexual desire in marriage? The most important are positive feelings about the spouse and anticipation of being sexual. The components of sexual desire are feeling good about yourself as a sexual person, believing you deserve sexual pleasure, and anticipating sex. Core sources include shared intimacy, affectionate and sensual touching both inside and outside the bedroom, experience of success on the job or athletically, completion of a house or other project with sex as a reinforcer. Sex can be anticipated as a tension reducer after a hard day; a movie, fantasy, or the sight of someone attractive promotes desire; sex as a way to compensate for a life defeat; a vacation with the freedom and privacy to play out sexual feelings. Sexual desire can and should come from a number of sources, especially feelings and anticipation.

BLOCKS TO SEXUAL DESIRE

Occasional lack of sexual desire is an almost universal phenomenon for both women and men, although men would not admit it. Stresses such as illness, job pressure, depression, lack of sleep, worry about children, grieving, money pressures, and anxiety result in inhibited desire. This is temporary—when the stress lifts, desire returns. Inhibited sexual desire is a problem only when it extends over a period of time and causes relationship stress.

Inhibited sexual desire (also called lack of libido or hypoactive sexual desire) is the most common complaint of couples seeking sex therapy. Approximately 33 percent of married women and 15 percent of married men complain of inhibited sexual desire. Over time desire problems become severe and chronic. Couples argue who is to blame for the lack of sexual contact. Conflicts over initiation and rejection loom large. These degenerate into power struggles filled with name-calling and blaming.

Couples plagued with inhibited desire focus on the wrong issue. They emphasize frequency; one partner tries to convince the other to have intercourse. A productive focus is improving quality of intimacy and sexuality rather than quantity of intercourse. Inhibited sexual desire is best conceptualized as a couple problem, which avoids putting pressure and blame on one spouse. If sex is to be comfortable, pleasurable and functional, the partners need to be a team in developing a couple sexual style which promotes and nurtures desire.

Even when one partner—usually the woman—reports primary inhibited sexual desire (she never thought of sex as a positive element in life and always had a low sex drive), it is a couple task to develop a satisfying sexual relationship. We encourage couples to seek therapy for inhibited sexual desire. Therapy helps them break the pattern of blame, guilt, and avoidance and learn to communicate and work as an intimate team. More than other sexual problems, inhibited desire brings out the worst in the partner, undermining the marriage. The spouse with higher desire sometimes blames himself, but most often blames the partner. He accuses her of being "frigid" and tries to convince or coerce her to be sexual. He might threaten to separate or have an affair. When it is the woman who has higher desire, she sees his lack of interest as a personal rejection or her lack of attractiveness. There is suspicion the spouse is having an affair or is gay. Self-blame and frustration is turned against the partner. Especially harmful is an attack on his masculinity or her femininity. This exacerbates the problem, leading to emotional alienation.

The spouse need not personalize inhibited sexual desire. It is important to maintain your own desire and sexual pleasure. Your sexual interest is a friend and booster for the relationship. If you develop a sexual dysfunction or inhibited desire, the problem is compounded.

SEXUAL DYSFUNCTION AND INHIBITED SEXUAL DESIRE

Which comes first, sexual dysfunction or inhibited desire? This is not the "chicken or egg" argument it might appear.

There are couples for whom sexual dysfunction—especially male erection and female orgasm problems—clearly preceded inhibited desire. Other couples have nonsexual stresses such as loss of a job, conflict over child management, illness, or obesity, which lowered desire, and subsequently one or both developed a sexual dysfunction. Stress from an extramarital affair or chronic marital conflict results in sexual problems, often inhibited desire. Perhaps the most common pattern is a couple who had a mediocre sexual relationship. Over time, sex became unsatisfactory, resulting in inhibited desire. The desire problem robs the couple of motivation and energy to deal with emotional and sexual issues.

Jill and Robert

Jill was pleased she hadn't fallen into the traditional female trap of not being aware of and valuing sex. As an adolescent, she discovered masturbation and was orgasmic at age fifteen. She enjoyed dating and petting, beginning intercourse at seventeen (this was the norm for Jill's peer group, although she hoped her daughter would delay intercourse until at least nineteen). Like many women, Jill found it easier to be orgasmic with manual and oral stimulation than intercourse. She enjoyed sex but disliked the roller coaster emotions inherent in dating relationships. A difficult experience for Jill was contracting chlamydia. She treated this as a medical issue not a moral one, and there were no long-term physical problems.

Jill expected sex to be a positive, exciting part of her life. She obtained an associate degree in office management and was working at a highly respected law firm. Her goal was to become an office manager.

Office affairs are discouraged in management manuals, but they occur with surprising frequency. Jill was attracted to Robert, who had recently been made a partner—she found him bright and witty. Robert's marriage was coming apart and Jill was there as a friend and emotional supporter. Not surprisingly, sexual attraction grew, and their relationship turned into an affair.

Jill enjoyed being with Robert, and found the sex exciting. However, she was put off because he didn't talk about sex as easily as other men she'd been with. Although he was easily

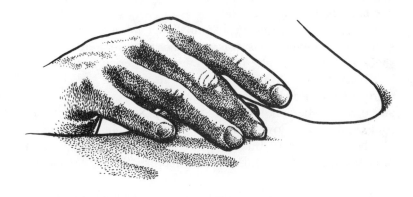

Anticipating and valuing pleasuring and sexuality is the best way
to maintain sexual desire.

aroused and orgasmic, he was not emotionally expressive or sexually playful. Jill was orgasmic, so wondered if she was making something out of nothing.

From Robert's perspective, sex was easy and straightforward. He'd begun masturbating at twelve, had his first partner orgasm petting in a car when a junior in high school, and first intercourse the summer before he entered college. Sexually, Robert functioned automatically and autonomously. In other words, he experienced desire, arousal, and orgasm with no need for help from his partner. The woman he began dating in his sophomore year was the person he married four years later while in law school. Robert was an ambitious, goal-directed person who took the marriage for granted. He found marital sex satisfactory, but frequency was erratic. When under stress he liked "quickie" intercourses to relieve tension.

Robert planned to begin a family after he achieved partner status, and assumed this was what his wife desired. He was shocked to discover she had an entirely different agenda. She had been having an affair for over two years and planned to marry this man and move overseas. Throughout the separation and divorce, she was hostile and cutting. She said Robert was egotistical, a poor lover, and clueless about feelings and needs of others. For Robert, Jill was a safe port in a tumultuous storm of attack and negation. Jill respected and liked Robert, assuaging his self-doubts.

Jill's involvement with Robert was not acceptable to the law firm. She left for a job as assistant office manager in the city's biggest, but badly managed, law firm. The change was a disaster for her career and later turned into a source of resentment in the marriage. A common cause of inhibited sexual desire is resentment over sacrifices made by the woman for the man's career.

Once Robert was assured Jill wanted to marry, he began to take the relationship for granted. This included routine, quick sex. Rather than sex improving with time as Jill had hoped, it fell into an unsatisfactory pattern. Yet Jill felt committed to Robert so stifled dissatisfaction.

The incident that accelerated the downhill cycle occurred on the wedding night. Jill was expecting a romantic, special experience. Instead, she got the same sex routine. She was furious and they had their worst fight ever. You are much better off arguing when you're clothed, sitting up, and not in the bedroom. In bed, especially after sex, there is a vulnerability that is easily elicited, with potentially long-term consequences. Robert felt unjustly attacked, which reminded him of feelings from his first marriage. Rather than talking with Jill, he retreated into a protective shell. This was the first and last sexual encounter of the honeymoon. It marked the beginning of Jill's inhibited sexual desire.

Jill regretted losing her temper, but felt Robert continuing to punish her was unfair. They were at a stalemate. Each felt like a wounded victim waiting for the other to apologize. The longer a stalemate continues, the harder it is to break, and the stronger are feelings of anger and resentment. Anger, more than any other emotion, subverts sexual desire. The time to deal with desire problems is within six months after they develop. Jill and Robert, like most couples, did not seek therapy until sexual avoidance and alienation had festered over many years.

The impetus for addressing the sexual problem was Jill's desire to have a child. It is difficult to conceive when you have intercourse less than once a month. Robert was reluctant to enter therapy because he was afraid he'd be blamed for the marital, sexual, and fertility problems. However, marital therapy is not about blame and refighting old battles. The goal of marital therapy is to revitalize the intimate bond and make the relationship satisfying for both people. After an initial couple session the clinician saw Jill and Robert individually, trying to understand the perceptions, feelings, and desires of each.

At the feedback session, the therapist emphasized how important it was for them to make a good faith commitment to revitalize their marital and sexual bond. She noted that it takes at least six months to develop a functional and satisfying couple sexual style. That process had been detoured by the incident on the honeymoon. They needed to work as an intimate team to communicate, increase comfort, reintroduce pleasuring, and create eroticism. Most important, they needed to be open to revitalizing intimacy and rebuilding bridges to desire.

Jill and Robert had a strong commitment to their marriage in spite of the sexual disappointments. Jill took her marital vows seriously. Robert did not want the stigma of being a "two-time loser." The desire to have a child and the excitement of trying to get pregnant can be a boon to sexual desire.

Although initially hesitant, Robert was willing to devote the time and psychological energy to revitalizing marital sex. He found it easy to reawaken desire, and took seriously Jill's request to improve the quality of marital sex. Jill found it difficult to build bridges to sexual desire. She had not expected to be in this situation, and needed to let go of anger and resentment before she could be truly desirous of Robert. Jill was surprised that her ability to be aroused and orgasmic was easier to regain than sexual desire. As intimacy, pleasuring, and erotic experiences continued, her trust in Robert grew. The excitement of trying to get pregnant increased Jill's desire.

During the pregnancy, Jill and Robert discussed the importance of maintaining emotional and sexual intimacy. The birth of a first child is a major transition in a couple's life. They were committed to maintaining their hard-won intimacy. Jill and Robert made a positive transition from being a couple to being a family.

PRIMARY INHIBITED SEXUAL DESIRE

Primary inhibited sexual desire is almost always a female problem. It's a direct result of our culture's attempts, directly and indirectly, to stifle female sexuality until marriage. Parental and societal admonitions against masturbation and sexual play, warnings about a woman's "reputation," avoiding pregnancy, concern about STDs and HIV, fear of rape, and vigilance about being taken advantage of has a more potent and lasting effect than anticipated. A young woman is not supposed to view herself as a sexual person nor value sexual expression. Being married does not magically cure this problem or remove the destructive sexual assumptions. Males do not suffer from primary inhibited desire because they are taught to value sexuality, masturbate to orgasm, and see sexuality as a part of their masculine identity. These same learning opportunities need to be open to women.

Karen

Karen was thirty-two and had been married three years. She was a bright, sophisticated woman who was aware of and able to express a range of emotions. However, in discussing her sexual history, it was evident that she suffered from primary inhibited sexual desire until her mid-twenties.

Karen grew up as a "good girl" She had a warm and close relationship with both parents, and was a more agreeable child than her two older brothers. Both brothers married early, one because of an unplanned pregnancy. Karen's mother encouraged her to attend college and delay marriage. Part of that message was to delay sexuality, which in itself is not problematic. However, Karen took it to the extreme of avoiding self-exploration and masturbation, staying away from touching except kissing and hand-holding, and remaining as sexually naive and inexperienced as possible. She was socially active in groups and was a "buddy" to males, but shut down romantic or sexual opportunities. She viewed her parents' marriage as distant and her mother as a nonsexual woman. They were better at parenting than being an intimate couple.

Karen hoped to "fall in love" when she completed college, but that was not to be. She planned to remain a virgin until marriage. That's easier to do if you marry at eighteen or twenty-one, but not realistic if you marry at twenty-nine. Karen naively hoped marriage and her husband would bestow sexual desire on her.

Karen had to increase awareness of herself as a sexual person. Desire resides first in the individual and is nurtured through the relationship. Karen's goal was to have an emotionally intimate and secure marriage. This goal is shared by men as well as women. As with other aspects of life, there is a process to go through to reach your goal. "Paying your dues" means learning about yourself, men, relationships, and sexuality. Some experiences were positive, others difficult and painful.

Karen met Derrick when she was twenty-eight, and they married a year later. The sexual relationship developed well because Karen had a better understanding of herself and sexuality than at twenty-one. She had learned three major things about sexual desire that would serve her well in the marriage. Sex works best when (1) her conditions for the relationship were met (she felt valued, trusted the partner, and was protected against unwanted pregnancy and STDs/HIV), (2) she was aware of sexual feelings and fantasies and was open and receptive to affectionate and sensual touching, and (3) the male viewed her as an attractive, sexual woman and was open to her sexual requests and guidance. As the marriage progressed, intimacy and sexuality became integrated. For Karen, as with other women, this is the basis for maintaining sexual desire in marriage.

Inhibited sexual desire used to be considered rare in our sex-oriented culture. However, recent research makes it clear that inhibited sexual desire is the most common couple problem. People, males especially, are reluctant to admit desire problems. It's more socially acceptable to have a specific sexual dysfunction than to admit, "I just don't feel like having sex."

Pat and Dan

Pat and Dan entered marriage therapy as a last resort. Their children were young adults who lived independently. With the house to themselves, they hoped their sex life, which had always been mediocre or worse, would improve.

They labeled the problem as solely Pat's. She had never been desirous of sex, although when on vacation, she was responsive and orgasmic. Pat's explanation was that with all the other things in life she did not have the time or energy to be sexually involved. On vacation, with the pressure off, she was responsive, but in day-to-day life sex was a low priority. Pat believed she was not a very sexual person. It did not bother her that Dan had occasional sexual flings. She did resent his paying a prostitute or spending money on dinner and a hotel room.

Dan felt he had tried everything and there was nothing more he could do. He told friends he had a "good wife in the house but a dud in the sack" and would lament his lot to women he met, in particular a woman at a massage parlor he frequented weekly. One of the reasons Dan consented to seeing a therapist was the economic argument that it was cheaper (as well as safer) to pay for therapy to improve marital sex than spend money on dinners, hotels, prostitutes, and massage parlors.

As is usually the case, the causes of Pat's inhibited desire were a combination of sexual and nonsexual issues. Pat felt it was not "right" to initiate sex or appear to need sex. When Dan talked about sex, it was with the attitude "the best sex is dirty sex." Pat wanted no part of that. She enjoyed dirty jokes and was good at telling sex jokes, but could not imagine herself talking about sex comfortably or integrating sexuality into her self-esteem. Dan inadvertently reinforced her negative sexual attitudes by his double-standard approach.

After two weeks of therapy, it became evident that Dan's attitudes were a major factor in Pat's inhibitions. Dan did not have a high opinion of women. Pat was an excellent mother and homemaker, but these qualities were not valued by him. Dan felt that since he brought home the larger paycheck, he was the most important person in the family. He ridiculed his son for doing woman's work and turning into a sissy because he enjoyed cooking. Pat never confronted Dan, but built up years of resentment. Marital roles were rigid and stereotyped. This carried into sex: initiation was exclusively Dan's. Sex was to satisfy his needs, Pat was a passive recipient. In sexual and nonsexual ways, Pat's desire was inhibited not only by her attitudes and experiences, but just as strongly by Dan's attitudes and actions.

In order to make a sexual breakthrough, it was necessary for Pat and Dan to focus on nonsexual aspects of the relationship, especially their rigid view of male-female roles. Anger is the major inhibitor of sexual desire. Pat, like many women of her generation, expressed anger by turning off sexually. Verbally expressing resentment in a nonsexual context is one way to free sexual energy. One of the best ways to prevent inhibited sexual desire is to deal with nonsexual issues as they arise, and keep them out of the bedroom. Sexuality is not a good medium to deal with hurt, anger, or resentment.

At first, Dan was defensive when being confronted with his chauvinism. As the therapist sensitized Dan to the fact that this approach subverted his marital sex life, he came to recognize his attitudes and actions as inappropriate and self-defeating. Pat read about female sexuality and became clearer in identifying the kinds of touch and stimulation she was receptive and responsive to. She did not want to be "worked on" by Dan, who at every moment was evaluating how aroused she was. Pat rebelled against Dan's demand that she have one orgasm, which was to occur during intercourse at the same time as his. In one set of sexual exercises, the couple refrains from intercourse and engages in a variety of sensual and sexual activities that facilitate pleasure and arousal. As the therapist predicted, Dan responded with anxiety and inhibition, whereas Pat was enthusiastic and orgasmic. This made it clear to them that the lack of desire was a couple problem, not solely, or even principally, Pat's. Belatedly, Dan realized he had a lot to learn about being in a sexually intimate marriage.

MALE INHIBITED SEXUAL DESIRE

It is not only women who lack desire and avoid sex. Although seldom admitted or discussed, men too suffer from inhibited sexual desire. Approximately fifteen percent of males in their middle years report inhibited desire. When couples cease sexual activity, it is because the man has low desire or is afraid he's lost the ability to function.

Males say they simply lose desire, blaming it on age or the "same old thing with the same partner." These are easy rationalizations, but are not the real cause. Closer to the truth is that the man isolates himself from warm, intimate feelings and takes his wife and marriage for granted. He is drained by the stress of his job, preoccupied by sports, financial, or household interests, and discounts the value of marital sex in the middle and later years. He puts little emotional or creative energy into the sexual relationship. Inhibited sexual desire is the outcome. Part of the problem is lack of awareness; the man does not recognize or accept changes in sexual functioning that come with aging. Because sex is no longer easy and automatic does not mean he has lost his ability to function or his sexual desire. He needs to be receptive and responsive to the spouse. Desire and arousal is a function of intimate, interactive sex.

Primary inhibited sexual desire is rare in males. Adolescent males learn to value sexual expression, engage in masturbation and view sexuality as integral to masculinity. Causes of primary inhibited desire are a paraphiliac (variant) arousal pattern, conflict regarding sexual orientation, or a sexual fear or secret that alienates him from the partner.

Secondary inhibited sexual desire is as common in males as females. The sexual socialization that served a man well in his younger years sabotages sexuality with aging. A male learns sexual desire and functioning in an automatic, autonomous manner. He feels desire, becomes aroused and erect, and experiences orgasm with little or no input from the woman. Sexual desire and functioning is easy and totally in his control; all she needs to do is be there. This attitude sets the stage for developing sexual dysfunction and inhibited desire as he ages, especially with marital sex.

The most frequent cause of male secondary inhibited desire is a sexual dysfunction. The most common sexual problem for young males is early ejaculation (also called premature or rapid ejaculation). Men attempt to deal with this by reducing arousal and avoiding partner stimulation, which is absolutely the wrong strategy. A healthy focus is building awareness and comfort while increasing give-and-take stimulation. The most common trap which leads to erection problems is engaging in "do it yourself" techniques for ejaculatory control. This interferes with arousal and causes him to lose erectile confidence.

Most males cease being automatic, autonomous performers in their mid-thirties or forties. Since sex is no longer easy and totally under his control, he feels vulnerable and unsure. Reduced comfort and confidence puts him on the slippery slope to sexual dysfunction and inhibited desire. He no longer anticipates being sexual and instead worries about performance. Sex is not fun and pleasurable, but a task to perform and worry about how well he's done. It becomes a performance-oriented spectator sport rather than an active, involved sharing of pleasure. There are increasing periods of sexual avoidance. The old myth that the longer you go without sex the "hornier" you get is untrue. The truth is, sexual avoidance feeds on itself. The more irregular the sex, the lower the desire. The sex hormone, testosterone, increases after a sexual experience. It is regularity, anticipation and pleasure that maintains sexual desire.

No matter how much he wants to, a man with inhibited sexual desire cannot take a magic pill which returns him to automatic, autonomous functioning. He has to develop a new way of thinking about and experiencing sexuality. The key element is awareness that sexual arousal comes *from* the couple interaction, not apart from it. You are responsible for your sexuality, but are no longer an autonomous sexual being. Sexual desire and arousal are tied to what is going on emotionally and erotically between you and your spouse. Rather than starting with a spontaneous erection and high levels of arousal, sexual functioning comes from intimacy, pleasuring and stimulation. You need not mourn the loss of easy, autonomous sexuality. You can celebrate the opportunity for intimate, give-and-take sexual expression. Sexual desire comes from anticipation and being an active, involved partner in the pleasuring and erotic process.

CLOSING THOUGHTS

Enhancing sexual desire is a couple task. Desire can and does come from diverse sources. Both spouses are motivated to enhance and nurture desire. Relationships in which each person is receptive to nondemand touching both inside and outside the bedroom, pleasuring need not end in intercourse, and the couple can share intimately in sexual and nonsexual contexts, allow multiple avenues to experience and express sexuality. The major aphrodisiac is an involved, aroused partner. Her desire and arousal facilitates your desire and arousal.

Inhibited sexual desire is the most common yet complex sexual dysfunction. If it lasts more than six months, we suggest seeking therapy because desire problems become severe and chronic. Frustration, blaming, and avoidance builds.

You deserve to feel good about yourself as a sexual person. Sexuality can play an integral role in energizing the marital bond. Sexual desire is not magic; it has to be nurtured and enhanced. Revitalizing sexual desire is a couple task, communicating and feeling like an intimate team.

13
DEALING WITH FEMALE SEXUAL DYSFUNCTION

Women have a right to sexual desire, arousal, orgasm and satisfaction. The biggest mistake is defining female sexuality narrowly and mechanically. Sex does *not* equal intercourse. Sexual satisfaction does *not* equal orgasm. The myth is that if women had orgasms, they would not have sexual complaints, intimacy problems, or lack of satisfaction. We are strong advocates for female orgasm, but it's not the end all or be all of female sexuality.

Sexual function includes desire (anticipating being sexual and feeling you deserve sexual pleasure), arousal (receptivity and responsitivity to genital stimulation resulting in feeling turned on and vaginal lubrication) orgasm (letting go and allowing high arousal to culminate in a climax), and satisfaction (feeling good about yourself, the spouse, and your intimate bond). The most common female sexual dysfunctions (in order of frequency):

1. Secondary inhibited sexual desire.
2. Primary inhibited sexual desire.
3. Secondary nonorgasmic response during partner sex.
4. Arousal dysfunction.
5. Painful intercourse.
6. Primary nonorgasmic response during partner sex.
7. Primary nonorgasmic response.
8. Vaginismus.

Primary sexual dysfunction means there's always been a problem (i.e., primary nonorgasmic response during partner sex means she has never been orgasmic with a partner, whether with manual, oral, rubbing or intercourse stimulation). Secondary dysfunction means she was sexually functional, but has become dysfunctional (i.e., secondary nonorgasmic response means she had been orgasmic but now is not).

It's crucial to resolve the dysfunction when that is the main factor inhibiting desire. For example, if the woman had a history of being sexually desirous, but develops pain during intercourse and secondary nonorgasmic response, these are the focus of treatment. Pain-free and orgasmic sex will result in increased desire. On the other hand, when the desire problem is primary and chronic (whether or not she experiences orgasm), desire is the focus of treatment. For many women, both desire and dysfunction issues need to be addressed.

As with desire problems, arousal and orgasm dysfunction are best considered a couple issue. The traditional trap was to label the woman "frigid." Fortunately, that term has fallen into disrepute. The "politically correct" explanation is to blame the partner: "males are selfish, lousy lovers." The old trap was to blame the woman; the new trap is to blame the man. It's a cop-out to label the woman frigid or the man a lousy lover. Blaming makes the problem worse.

The therapeutic strategy is the one-two combination where the woman increases awareness and takes responsibility for her sexuality and the couple communicates and works as an intimate team. She takes an active, involved role in the pleasuring process. Key to arousal are receptivity and responsivity to erotic stimulation. She communicates and guides the spouse (either by putting her hand over his or making verbal requests), showing him what she prefers. They learn to talk, feel, and solve problems as an intimate team. He is open to her requests and guidance instead of playing the "macho" role of the sex expert. They are trusting, equitable partners.

In the traditional scenario the woman remains passive while the man "services" her during foreplay to get her ready for the main event of intercourse. Although some women prefer this scenario, the majority prefer "pleasuring." Pleasuring refers to giving and receiving sensual and sexual touching. They are an intimate team, enjoying each other's pleasure and arousal. One's arousal builds on the other's. The husband is an involved, caring partner. Pleasure and arousal are good in and of themselves, they do not have to be goal-oriented (i.e., leading to intercourse). Unfortunately, our culture labels erection as the measure of male sexuality and orgasm as the measure of female sexuality. These rigid performance criteria inhibit rather than facilitate sexual functioning and satisfaction.

There are massive misunderstandings about female arousal and orgasm. Old myths involved female passivity and less sexual capacity. Women felt pressure to be like men—have one orgasm during intercourse. Old myths have given way to new, performance-oriented myths. These include women must have an orgasm each time; orgasm is the only measure of satisfaction, primacy of the "G" spot, being multiorgasmic is superior to one orgasm.

The scientifically valid concept is female sexual response is variable, flexible and complex. Male response is predictable and stereotyped (i.e., he has one orgasm during intercourse). The woman can be singly orgasmic, nonorgasmic, or multiorgasmic, which can occur in the pleasuring/foreplay period, through intercourse, or during afterplay. Female sexual response is variable and flexible (this does not mean better or worse).

There is not "one right way" to experience orgasm. Only one in four women follow the male model of a single orgasm during intercourse. The most common pattern for "Jane and Joe Average" is Jane is orgasmic with manual and/or oral stimulation during pleasuring and Joe is orgasmic with intercourse. Many women can be orgasmic during intercourse, but find it easier to be orgasmic with nonintercourse sex. Most women do not have an orgasm at each sexual experience. Approximately twenty percent of women have a multiorgasmic response pattern. If she has six orgasms, does that mean she is six times more satisfied? There is no evidence that women who are multiorgasmic feel more sexually satisfied than women who are singly orgasmic. The woman develops an arousal and orgasm pattern which enhances her sexuality.

What does this mean for desire, arousal, orgasm and satisfaction? The key is understanding, accepting, and enjoying the variability and flexibility of female sexuality. Competing with a male performance standard subverts female sexuality. Each woman and couple develop their sexual response pattern—differences and preferences are respected and accepted. The woman is the expert on her sexuality, not the man nor an arbitrary performance criterion.

ORGASM DURING INTERCOURSE

Freud made the distinction between "vaginal orgasm," which he labeled as mature, normal and occurring during intercourse, and "clitoral orgasm," which occurred during self-stimulation or partner manual, oral, or rubbing stimulation. Freud labeled clitoral orgasm as immature, less than normal. Scientific research by Masters and Johnson and clinical work by sex therapists found this to be totally inaccurate. A rigid performance criterion is scientifically incorrect and psychologically self-defeating.

Physiologically, an orgasm is an orgasm—whether from masturbation, partner manual stimulation, intercourse, cunnilingus, vibrator stimulation, or rubbing stimulation. There are differences in women's preferences and satisfaction. The woman develops an arousal and orgasm pattern she feels comfortable and satisfied with. This may or may not include being orgasmic during intercourse.

Nonorgasmic response during intercourse is *not* a sexual dysfunction—it is a normal variation of female sexuality. If she is aroused and orgasmic during partner sex and enjoys intercourse, this is optimal for her. There is nothing "better" or "more mature" about orgasm during intercourse. Some women are orgasmic during intercourse with multiple stimulation—her own or partner manual clitoral stimulation, vibrator stimulation, or intercourse positions and movements which indirectly provide clitoral stimulation. If this is satisfying, that's great. It's neither superior nor inferior to women who are orgasmic through manual, oral, or rubbing stimulation. It's neither superior nor inferior to women who are orgasmic through intercourse stimulation alone. Orgasm is not a competitive performance. Orgasm is a natural result of involvement, pleasure, arousal, erotic flow, and emotionally and sexually letting go.

Let us examine in detail the most common arousal and orgasm dysfunctions.

SECONDARY NONORGASMIC RESPONSE DURING PARTNER SEX

This dysfunction has dramatically increased in the last decade and is a major cause of inhibited sexual desire. She had been orgasmic during partner sex, but no longer is or is rarely so (less than twenty percent). Part of the problem is performance anxiety and unrealistic expectations caused by the culture's emphasis on the "big O." Orgasm has received inordinate focus, more than any other aspect of female sexuality. It's as if female sexuality equals orgasm. It's become a measure of the man to ensure she has an orgasm. This performance focus is self-defeating and increases female secondary dysfunction.

Orgasm is integral to the comfort-pleasure-arousal cycle, not separate from it. Orgasm is the natural culmination of involved, effective sexual stimulation. Women have fallen into the male trap of pressuring themselves to be orgasmic each time, and, if not, feeling sex was a failure. You don't need the "right" orgasm to prove something to yourself or your spouse. Orgasm is an erotic flowing process. It begins with being aware of and responsible for your sexuality, receptive and responsive to stimulation, open to erotic scenarios and techniques, and letting go and allowing high arousal to flow into orgasm. Responsibility includes making sexual requests and guiding the partner. Your spouse cannot make you have an orgasm, nor is he responsible for your orgasm. He is caring, cooperative, and sharing—your intimate partner.

The most common causes of secondary nonorgasmic response are performance anxiety, anger, and emotional alienation. Sexual causes are easier to deal with than emotional inhibitions or conflicts. The sexual strategy is to increase comfort, pleasure and arousal while decreasing performance pressure. This begins with nondemand pleasuring and a temporary prohibition on orgasm and intercourse. Put play, pleasuring, and intimacy back into sexuality. Nondemand pleasuring and sensuality is the underpinning of sexual arousal.

Allow sensual and sexual touching to move at the woman's pace rather than the man's. She makes requests and he is open to her guidance. For example, some women prefer beginning genital touching with breast stimulation, others with vulva stimulation. This is not a matter of right or wrong—identify your receptivity-responsivity pattern(s) and share it with your spouse. Most women prefer indirect rather than direct clitoral stimulation. A common female complaint is that the male tires of rhythmic stimulation and does stimulation according to his desires. This breaks her arousal rhythm. The strategy for dealing with this dilemma is communicating your requests and utilizing multiple stimulation. Arousal involves maintaining rhythmic clitoral stimulation while adding erotic stimulation, which can include manual or oral breast stimulation, stimulation of the mons or anal area, kissing and caressing, intravaginal finger stimulation, vibrator stimulation, rubbing his penis against her breasts or vulva. Some women enjoy passively accepting stimulation, most prefer actively giving and receiving stimulation. Examples of being active include touching and stimulating him, focusing on a sexual fantasy, moving your body rhythmically to increase sensations, giving and receiving oral stimulation simultaneously, being in a standing or kneeling position, which heightens eroticism and allows rhythmic movement. Increasing involvement and eroticism is key.

Letting go and allowing arousal to flow into orgasm involves multiple factors. Especially where problems are caused by emotional and relationship inhibitions, the couple has to communicate and work as an intimate team. The change process is complex, undermined by miscommunication, misunderstandings and frustration. When these are the predominant causes, you are strongly encouraged to seek sex therapy.

Anger, more than anxiety, interferes with sexual expression. The woman who has turned off sexually because of anger or alienation finds it difficult to think of herself as on the same intimate team. Anger is a powerful inhibitor of sexual desire. Negative emotions such as depression, boredom, sadness, frustration, irritation, feeling put off, block sexual response. Relational factors such as lack of couple time, conflict about money, irritation concerning personal habits, disappointment in the spouse or marriage, repeating negative patterns from the family of origin, and conflict over intimacy inhibit sexual desire. Situational factors such as lack of privacy, phone ringing, kids coming in, no lock on the bedroom door, an uncomfortable bed, no time to be sexual, work stress, abuse of drugs or alcohol, side effects of antidepressant or other medications, interfere with sexual response. Making the psychological, relational, and situational changes necessary to enjoy arousal and orgasm is doable, but not simple. The couple loses motivation and focus. Professional intervention is recommended because the therapist helps you maintain focus and motivation. The longer the dysfunction exists, the more likely it will result in inhibited sexual desire.

Lily and Robert

It is not unusual that both partners have a problem with orgasm. A common pattern is the man is an early ejaculator and the woman is nonorgasmic during intercourse. This was the situation for Lily and Robert, a couple in their early thirties who had been married four years. Robert had always been an early ejaculator, but this had not concerned him. He thought of sex as intercourse, and saw himself as a lusty, passionate male. Lily had been orgasmic, although infrequently, with other partners. Initially she enjoyed Robert's sexual passion, but became disillusioned even before they married.

Robert was very intercourse-oriented, spending less than five minutes on foreplay, which was mechanical and perfunctory. He was erect and ready to go before his clothes were off. It wasn't just ejaculation that was rapid, it was his whole approach to sex. Males who have spontaneous erections and early ejaculation do not want to be stimulated, because they mistakenly believe it speeds ejaculation. Lily saw Robert as a selfish partner, uninterested in her sexual feelings and needs. He was worried because Lily wasn't sexually interested or orgasmic. His reaction was to be more intense and intercourse-focused, which only compounded the problem.

Lily made the classic sexual mistake. After intercourse, she expressed her frustration, which caught Robert off guard. His defensiveness quickly became offensive. They had a half-hour yelling-and-crying match, blaming, calling names, and "hitting below the belt." Robert called Lily "frigid" and a loser. Lily called Robert a "pig" and the worse lover she'd ever had. You are very vulnerable when nude and lying in bed. It is the wrong time to voice frustrations or sexual complaints. It's easy for this to get out of control and degenerate into a "pissing contest." The only good thing that came out of the debacle was a decision to seek therapy rather than allow the marriage to degenerate.

A key concept in sex therapy is to view the dysfunction as a couple problem and avoid the guilt-blame cycle. The issue is not

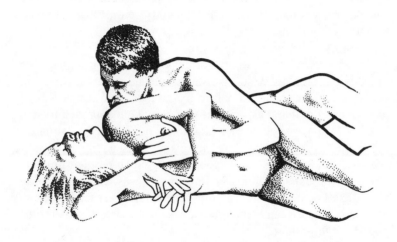

Orgasm is a natural response to heightened sexual arousal and psychologically letting go.

blame—arguing whether the partner caused or didn't cause the problem. The key point is working together to develop a couple sexual style that is comfortable, functional, and satisfying. As Barry says during therapy, "Sex is a team sport—you support the mate, don't turn on her."

Lily and Robert felt relieved they were addressing sexual concerns in a constructive manner. In conducting individual histories, it was apparent that Robert had shifted from being unaware to feeling the whole burden was on him, specifically to make Lily have an orgasm during intercourse. Moving from one extreme to another is a mistake. Robert believed it was his responsibility to make Lily respond just like him, and have a single orgasm during intercourse. To accomplish this he thought all he needed was to prolong intercourse for thirty minutes. The therapist explained this was a self-defeating way to view ejaculatory control. Sex was not a performance he gave to win Lily's orgasm. Robert would learn ejaculatory control for himself, increase awareness and comfort, and enjoy a range of pleasurable sensations, especially long, slow thrusting. Robert was responsible for ejaculatory control, and needed Lily's active involvement in the learning process.

Lily was responsible for increasing awareness and orgasmic response, and needed Robert's active involvement. Lily's sexual pattern had been to follow the man's direction. Most of her premarital partners had been like Robert, intercourse-oriented. Two of the men had spent time attending to her sexual needs. One used a variety of stimulation positions, and Lily was highly aroused. However, as soon as he felt she was ready, he moved to intercourse. The other man was insecure about erections, and preferred manual and oral stimulation. He was the partner with whom Lily had the most orgasms, but she tired of working so hard to get him aroused and was put off by his avoidance of intercourse.

Lily liked Robert's enthusiasm for intercourse, but missed manual and oral stimulation. She had been too embarrassed to make those requests. Lily had to be active and aware, take responsibility for arousal and orgasm, and give up the fantasy that all she needed was for Robert to maintain ejaculatory control.

The couple feedback session was particularly helpful in giving Lily and Robert an understanding of the problem and a way to approach change as a cooperative, intimate team. Especially important was the concept of each person assuming responsibility for his/her sexual awareness and functioning. Robert did not see the value of starting with nongenital pleasuring, but after the first three exercises he was a convert. The idea of slowing down and enjoying pleasuring was important, but of special value was openness to receiving stimulation. For Lily, taking initiatives, especially developing pleasuring scenarios and guiding Robert in what was arousing for her, was of particular value.

A serendipitous effect of sex therapy is that some women learn a multiorgasmic response pattern. Lily discovered sexual scenarios which were highly arousing. She enjoyed Robert combining oral breast stimulation with manual clitoral stimulation, while she rhythmically moved her pelvis. She particularly enjoyed a pleasuring position where she was standing and he kneeling, stimulating her breasts manually while orally stimulating her vulva. Switching intercourse positions greatly increased Lily's arousal, particularly combined with multiple stimulation. Lily was pleased to discover that when she was involved and creative, orgasm was easy.

Robert found sex therapy more difficult than Lily. This is not unusual, for women are more open and receptive to the permission-giving and experimentation components of sex therapy than men. Lily blossomed under the exploratory context of the sexual exercises. Robert learned and experienced new things, but was distracted by worries about sexual performance. He found it difficult to let go and fully enjoy the pleasuring process. It was hard for him to be in a position where he needed help from Lily. This is the heart of sexual intimacy, seeing the spouse as your intimate friend and being open to giving and receiving pleasuring and responsive to requests and guidance.

Intercourse was reintroduced as part of the pleasuring process via the quiet vagina exercise. This entailed Lily guiding intromission from the woman on top position, with minimal movement. The experience of having Robert inside her for five to ten minutes and feeling the sensations of intravaginal containment was good for Lily, but not erotic. Realizing he could be in the vagina that long was reinforcing. Learning ejaculatory control is a gradual process. It involves experimenting with different types and rhythms of thrusting and intercourse positions.

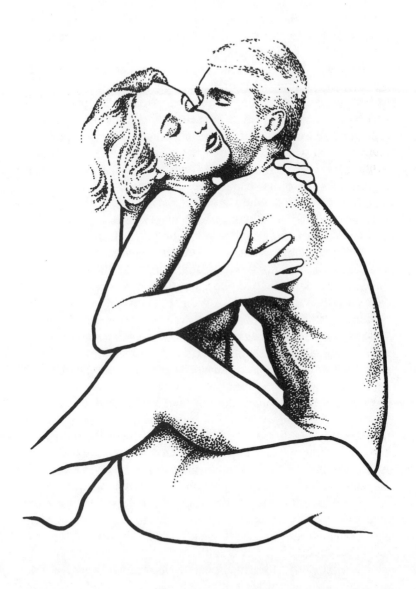

You cannot will or force arousal. Sexual arousal comes from receptivity and responsivity to stimulation.

AROUSAL DYSFUNCTION

For many women the problem is not orgasm, but arousal. Her subjective and objective arousal is low or nonexistent. Subjective arousal refers to feeling involved and turned on. Objective arousal includes vaginal lubrication, increased muscle tension, blood flow to the vulva, nipples becoming hard. Some women are orgasmic at low levels of arousal, but typically arousal flows to high levels, culminating in orgasm. Arousal dysfunction can be primary, but more often is secondary. A common theme is higher arousal in premarital than marital sex. Some women feel more aroused when clothes are on. Others say sex was more fun in the back seat of the car. The over-focus on intercourse and orgasm robs sex of its seductiveness, playfulness, and creativity.

A key to understanding arousal dysfunction is the different sexual socialization of women and men. Males typically learn arousal and orgasm through masturbation. Men learn that arousal is easy, predictable, automatic. He gets spontaneous erections, arousal is autonomous—he needs nothing from the woman. Female arousal is interactive, variable, slower, and can be lost because of distracting stimuli. Women learn to masturbate to orgasm in childhood or during adolescence. However, for many women, masturbation begins later or doesn't occur. Interestingly, rates of female masturbation increase with marriage. A significant number of women are unsure of their arousal pattern. It is hard to share if you're not aware yourself.

Experiences with manual, oral, and rubbing stimulation are unsatisfactory. She reacts to his sexual style and needs rather than establishing her own. The rhythm of touching is his, not hers. Very few women experience autonomous sexual arousal. Arousal is an interactive, intimate experience involving receptivity and responsivity to stimulation. The most common sexual blocks are too little time in pleasuring and poor stimulation techniques. Rather than blaming the spouse, labeling him as an uncaring and insensitive lover, she takes responsibility. This includes awareness of her conditions for good sex—psychologically, relationally, and situationally. One woman's arousal dramatically increased after asking the husband to put a lock on their bedroom door, brush his teeth before kissing, and being sexual between 7 and 7:30 in the morning. For some women, a prime condition for good sex is feeling emotionally close before beginning touching. For others, kissing and touching promotes intimacy. For some, talking facilitates arousal—for others, talking distracts from arousal. Be aware of your conditions for arousing sex and communicate these.

Your sexual feelings and needs are as important as his. When there is an arousal dysfunction, the couple is better to follow her rhythm of touching and stimulation. The major mistake men make as arousal builds is to increase the speed and hardness of stimulation. He does this not to subvert her arousal, but because that is his arousal pattern. She needs to communicate her rhythm of arousal. The most common pattern is regular, slow, gradually building erotic stimulation. Some women prefer to focus on one form of stimulation at a time. The majority prefer multiple stimulation. Some prefer receiving, others find give-and-take stimulation most arousing. Many women find stimulating the spouse arousing. Be aware of your psychological, relational, erotic, and situational preferences. Make clear, specific requests. Communicating as an intimate team facilitates arousal.

Lauren and Nathan

Lauren and Nathan had been a couple for sixteen years and married for eight. They were in their late thirties and had two children under five. Nathan was always the sexual initiator. He would stimulate Lauren to increase arousal but himself had spontaneous erections. She was used to the passive role and being given to. Nathan enjoyed the active role of giver. The expectation was that Nathan would be ready and willing for sex any time Lauren was.

The male-female double standard might work for couples in their twenties, but causes trouble when couples reach their thirties; few couples in their forties find it useful. As they age, men and women become more alike sexually. This results in better sex if the transition is understood and accepted. Expectations based on the male-female double standard have to dramatically change. At its best, sexuality is mutual sharing, an intimate giving and receiving of pleasure. Since a man no longer functions automatically and autonomously (usually beginning in the mid-thirties to early forties), he learns to be open to her stimulation. The woman can initiate, be sexually active, and enjoy a range

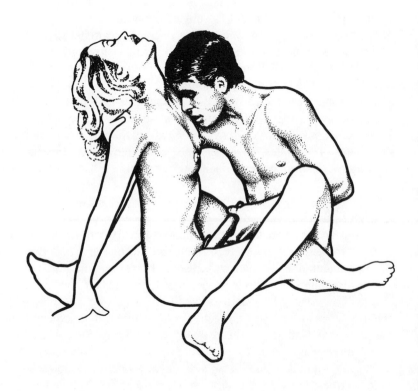

Vibrator stimulation can enhance arousal before or during intercourse.

of sexual scenarios and techniques instead of remaining stuck in the passive role.

Lauren found this an easier transition than Nathan. She genuinely enjoyed initiating sex play. It was intriguing to realize that she could excite him with her hands and tongue. Arousing Nathan was arousing for Lauren. Nathan discovered that an involved, aroused partner is a major sexual aphrodisiac.

PAINFUL INTERCOURSE

Painful intercourse (the technical term is dyspareunia) occurs on occasion to the great majority of women. It is a chronic problem for ten to fifteen percent. Consult a gynecologist for a comprehensive assessment of hormonal, vascular, neurological, and structural causes of painful intercourse. If a specific physical cause is not found, the woman concludes it's all in her head and feels put down. Pain is real; it's a complex psychophysiological process. Often, the best way to deal with painful intercourse is through psychological and behavioral changes rather than medication or surgery.

Two techniques are especially valuable for reducing or avoiding pain during intromission. The first is for the woman to initiate and guide intromission. This makes sense, since she is the expert on her vagina. The second is to use a lubricant to facilitate intromission and coital thrusting. Many women use K-Y Jelly because it's a sterile substance they're familiar with from gynecological exams. Other women prefer lubricants which feel or smell sensuous—be sure they are hypoallergenic and water-based to prevent infection. Favorites are Astroglide, abalone lotion, baby oil, aloe vera lotion, or flavored lotions. This is especially helpful for women who feel aroused, but have limited lubrication. There are a number of causes of decreased lubrication, including aging. Forty-year-old women lubricate less than twenty-year-old women, and sixty-year-old women lubricate less than forty-year-old women.

A common cause of painful intercourse is discomfort resulting from prolonged coital thrusting. The average time spent in intercourse is 2–7 minutes (the average time for the entire lovemaking experience is 15 to 45 minutes). Less than 10 percent of intercourse extends longer than 10 minutes. Women who are orgasmic during nonintercourse sex still enjoy intercourse. However, her involvement and arousal will decrease after 10 minutes of thrusting, as vaginal irritation increases. Especially if he engages in hard, prolonged thrusting, she is in danger of irritation, which can be painful as well as heighten the risk of tearing the vaginal walls and/or developing an infection. It's important that she communicate when discomfort begins to avoid pain.

One way to increase involvement and arousal is multiple stimulation during intercourse. Why should kissing, caressing, playful touching, erotic stimulation stop when the penis enters the vagina? Touching during intercourse can include breast stimulation, buttock stimulation, clitoral stimulation, testicle stimulation. Switch intercourse positions or types of stroking if there is discomfort. Many women find circular thrusting particularly pleasurable or enjoy long, slow thrusting. Men prolong intercourse with the hope the woman will reach orgasm, not realizing she's not turned on. Sexual communication is crucial.

There are a number of gynecological interventions for difficult, complex, or chronic cases. The most intrusive is surgery. Alternatives include exercises to strengthen vaginal muscles, suppositories, and medications. Be sure you have a good rapport with your gynecologist and she takes your problem seriously. Referral to a subspecialist in gynecological pain might be advisable. Ask your spouse to accompany you to appointments. Be clear on how he can be supportive in dealing with painful intercourse.

PRIMARY NONORGASMIC DYSFUNCTION—BY SELF AND WITH PARTNER

Primary nonorgasmic dysfunction also called preorgasmic) means the woman has never experienced orgasm by any means (5–10 percent of adult women). The more common problem is primary nonorgasmic dysfunction during partner sex (10–15 percent). She is orgasmic with self or vibrator stimulation, but not during partner sex. Approximately half of young women learn to be orgasmic during masturbation, the other half with partner manual, oral, or rubbing stimulation. Less than 10 percent have their first orgasm during intercourse.

The treatment of choice for preorgasmic women involves increased sexual awareness, body exploration, and masturbation. This can be done individually, augmented by self-help materials and exercises, or through a ten-session women's sexuality group. The group reduces stigma, provides practical and emotional support, and motivation for change as you see others progressing. Masturbation as a treatment technique was revolutionary a generation ago—professionals had argued whether masturbation was normal. Self-exploration and masturbation is now recognized as the easiest way of learning to be orgasmic. Men have few problems reaching orgasm, in part because of masturbation.

The woman who is aware of her arousal and orgasm pattern can transfer this knowledge to partner sex. Masturbation promotes a healthy, self-affirming attitude toward your body and taking responsibility for sexuality. Use of vibrator stimulation as an adjunct to masturbation has become popular in the past twenty years. The speed and intensity of vibrator stimulation breaks down inhibitions and self-consciousness and serves as an orgasm trigger. Although women fear becoming "hooked" on the vibrator, most find the transition to hand or rubbing stimulation easy. She uses vibrator stimulation (either alone or during partner sex) as a special turn-on.

The woman is aware of and uses "orgasm triggers" with masturbation. These techniques facilitate moving from high levels of arousal to orgasm. Orgasm triggers are variable and individualistic. They include tightening leg and/or thigh muscles to build tension until it bursts forth in orgasm, verbalizing that you're "going to come," doing breast and clitoral stimulation simultaneously as you move toward orgasm, using vibrator or intravaginal finger stimulation to enhance orgasmic sensations. Erotic stimulation is focused and rhythmic. Once you've identified orgasm triggers, transfer these to partner sex.

For many women, the transition to orgasm with a partner is easy, for others, difficult. If nonorgasmic response during partner sex involves a specific sexual inhibition, it is simpler to resolve than if there is an emotional inhibition. The most direct technique is stimulating yourself to orgasm with the spouse present. Sexually and emotionally this is a major breakthrough. He observes how she becomes aroused and reaches orgasm (which is motivating and exciting). Then, he (with her guidance) stimulates her to orgasm. For women who feel self-conscious, asking him to be vulnerable and do it first can be freeing.

A key concept is that the woman has a right to take the sexual lead, make requests, and set an erotic rhythm. He is open and responsive to her requests. It's important to discard the belief that it's his responsibility to "make her come." This pressure wilts her desire and arousal. The pressure on him results in frustration and anger, which negates his role as an involved, intimate spouse. Neither she nor he can force orgasm.

Orgasm is a natural result of erotic stimulation and letting go. Orgasm cannot be willed, forced, or coerced. Focus on the positions, feelings, and erotic techniques which heighten arousal. If you think of arousal on a scale of 0 (neutral) to 5 (moderate) to 10 (orgasm), most women find the problem in progressing from 0 to 5. Neither cunnilingus nor intercourse is arousing unless feelings are at least 5 and preferably a 7 before beginning these activities. Otherwise, it is counterproductive, resulting in self-consciousness.

Typically, couples transition into intercourse at the man's initiative when he feels she's ready. Let the woman initiate when to begin intercourse or cunnilingus. Many women find it easier to be orgasmic with oral stimulation. Being orgasmic is more than prolonging stimulation. Moving from 5 to 8 on the arousal scale involves making verbal and nonverbal requests to enhance eroticism. These include multiple stimulation such as combining manual clitoral stimulation, oral breast stimulation, and stroking his penis; closing your eyes and involving yourself in an erotic fantasy as you enjoy cunnilingus; switching positions to kneeling or standing while moving your body in rhythm with his stimulation; rubbing your clitoris against his penis or thigh while he is playing with your breasts or buttocks. Use of orgasm triggers allows arousal to flow from 8 to 10. Orgasm triggers in partner sex are the same as or similar to orgasm triggers with masturbation.

Some women prefer or need intercourse for orgasm. Sexuality and sexual response is about individual differences. Starting intercourse at level 5, or preferably 7, facilitates arousal during intercourse. Let the woman set the rhythm of thrusting—this is easier in the woman on top or side intercourse positions. Use of additional clitoral stimulation by her hand, his hand, or vibrator allows arousal to build toward orgasm. Asking him to make specific movements or putting your hands on his buttocks and guiding his movements is a valuable technique. Communicate and experiment to develop an arousal pattern which allows you to be orgasmic during partner sex.

VAGINISMUS

This is an infrequent sexual dysfunction, but one which disrupts the relationship and drains desire. Vaginismus refers to the tightening or spasming of the vaginal introitus, making intercourse impossible or very painful. A gynecological examination is necessary for diagnosis. Vaginismus requires sex therapy using *in vivo* desensitization (often with use of vaginal dilators). Active involvement and support of the spouse is crucial. The good news is the likelihood of successful treatment is high, the bad news is it's a gradual, sometimes frustrating, process. Maintaining motivation and working as an intimate team is critical, but can be emotionally taxing. Couples do best when they're open to non-intercourse sensual and sexual experiences. This maintains a bridge to sexual desire and feeling physically and emotionally connected. Couples who stop physical contact are faced with the double task of rebuilding connection and confronting vaginismus.

Often the impetus which motivates the couple is a desire to become pregnant. The need for intravaginal ejaculation challenges the pattern of avoidance. Although gynecologists do insemination with the husband's sperm, most couples prefer trying to become pregnant naturally, i.e., through intercourse. Desire for a child is a powerful motivator. The couple works as an intimate team using the resources of a gynecologist and sex therapist. She increases awareness and control of vaginal muscles, and gradually guides intromission. They use woman-on-top intercourse with slow, comfortable thrusting. One benefit of treating vaginismus is, it increases the woman's awareness, responsibility, and valuing of sexuality, which inoculates her against sexual problems in the future.

Faith and Sam

Faith and Sam had been married four and a half years. They were convinced they were the only couple in America who had been married that long and not consummated the marriage. Faith's vaginismus had been diagnosed by the gynecologist before marriage, but he had not made a recommendation for treatment. The minister who married them counseled love and support, but said nothing specific about sex. In their premarital life Faith and Sam had been a sexually active and functional couple utilizing oral and rubbing stimulation. This decreased over time. Faith developed secondary arousal dysfunction, secondary orgasmic dysfunction, and secondary inhibited sexual desire. Sam remained sexually functional, but was hostile and emotionally distant. He'd had two one-night affairs and threatened an ongoing affair. Faith felt that would be devastating and throw the marriage into crisis. She had sex with Sam one to two times a week, but it was one way-sex, where she "serviced" him. These experiences further reduced Faith's desire. Sam enjoyed orgasm, but felt emotionally isolated. It was a self-defeating cycle which protected them from addressing desire, arousal, orgasm, and vaginismus problems.

The motivation which led to sex therapy was a shared desire to become pregnant. Sam viewed this as a bond which would hold the marriage together (a questionable rationale, but helpful for Sam and Faith). Children were an integral part of Faith's life plan, and she was strongly motivated to resolve her vaginismus and become pregnant. The gynecologist recommended bypassing the sexual issue by using artificial insemination with Sam's sperm. Neither was enthusiastic about that technological solution, so he made a referral to a female sex therapist with expertise in treating vaginismus.

Sam and Faith were relieved to learn that other couples have nonconsummated marriages, and that vaginismus is a treatable problem with a good prognosis. The fact that Faith's desire, arousal, and orgasm dysfunctions were secondary showed she had the potential to enjoy sex. Inadvertently, Sam's sexual attitudes and behavior exacerbated Faith's dysfunction. Sam was surprised when the therapist asked if he wanted to be Faith's intimate friend or her sexual critic (the role he now played). Desire had been subverted by frustration, they'd been working at cross-purposes. Each had to take responsibility for his/her sexual behavior. Sam had to begin thinking, acting, and feeling like an intimate spouse.

With Faith taking the initiative, Sam being the intimate friend who enjoyed giving, and performance pressure reduced, desire was reignited. The transition to outercourse for arousal and orgasm was not difficult. Viewing erotic videos and Sam verbalizing sexual fantasies significantly enhanced Faith's arousal. At a different time, they did the slow, painstaking exercises to confront vaginismus. Faith learned physical relaxation techniques, specific pelvic relaxation, pubococcygeal muscle control, use of dilators for vaginal insertion, movement with fingers and dilators, and playing with Sam's penis around her vagina. Faith felt in control of the process, proceeding gradually, reducing fear and discomfort. Sam was her active supporter and "cheerleader."

Once intromission occurred, they didn't immediately go to intercourse but became accustomed to intravaginal sensations. Faith had to experience intercourse as functional before she could perceive it as pleasurable. Luckily, they were a couple who easily became pregnant (at their fourth month of trying). Faith didn't begin enjoying intercourse until six months after the baby was born. Sam and Faith were satisfied with their lovemaking style, which integrated manual, oral and intercourse stimulation.

CLOSING THOUGHTS

A woman learns to value sexuality for herself and the marriage. The bad news is, rates of sexual dysfunction are higher for women than men. The good news is successful resolution of sexual problems is easier for women. Women do better in and feel they get more from couples sex therapy. There is not a direct relationship between sexual function and sexual desire. Usually both issues have to be addressed, as well as the broader issue of intimacy.

14

DEALING WITH MALE SEXUAL DYSFUNCTION

Do desire problems cause sexual dysfunction or does sexual dysfunction cause desire problems? For the great majority of males, the causation is clear—sexual dysfunction eventually results in inhibited sexual desire. The major male sexual dysfunctions are early ejaculation, erectile dysfunction, and ejaculatory inhibition. For males, desire problems are almost always secondary. In other words, he's been desirous, but is now inhibited. The pattern is anticipatory anxiety, performance anxiety resulting in dysfunctional sex, and sexual avoidance due to embarrassment and failure.

Males learn desire, arousal, and orgasm as something that comes easy and automatic. The great majority of males masturbate by age sixteen, usually beginning between ten to fourteen. The combination of masturbatory orgasms and masculinity and sexuality being so closely associated reinforces sexual desire for the adolescent and young adult male. This pattern has value, but poses vulnerabilities with dysfunction or aging. Ease and quantity of youthful sex is not a solid basis for adult male sexuality. For example, an eighteen-year-old ejaculates, has a short latency period before he is receptive to stimulation, and then has another orgasm. Is this the best measure of male sexual functioning or satisfaction? The easy, automatic, autonomous, quantity approach to sexuality sets the stage for sexual dysfunction as you age.

By their mid-thirties or early forties most men find arousal is no longer autonomous, they now need partner stimulation. About one in three men finds this transition difficult and develops desire or arousal problems. Emphasizing sexual frequency rather than quality is self-defeating. The focus on performance rather than pleasure makes him vulnerable to dysfunction. The worst thing one can believe is that sexual autonomy is better than intimate, interactive sex. Over time, especially in marriage, intimacy is a key bridge to maintaining sexual desire. Our prescription for sexual satisfaction is intimacy, nondemand pleasuring and eroticism. Male sexual socialization emphasizes only the last component.

A common male fear (which becomes a self-fulfilling prophecy) is that if he loses self-confidence and goal orientation, he'll enter a "slippery slope" of being sexually self-conscious and losing erections. In other words, the cycle of positive anticipation, enjoying intercourse and orgasm, and frequent sex disappears. It is replaced by anticipatory anxiety, tense and increasingly failed intercourse, and sexual avoidance. What accounts for this self-defeating cycle? Self-consciousness, distraction, and performance anxiety. Sex is an active, involved, participatory activity—not a spectator sport. There is an erotic flow where each spouse's desire, receptivity, and responsibility enhances the other's. This is the basis of the "give to get" pleasuring guideline. At the core sexuality is pleasure-oriented touching. The spouse being "turned on" is a turn-on for you. Distraction and self-consciousness break the erotic flow, resulting in lowered arousal. When sex becomes a pass-fail performance, you have created conditions for failure and sexual dysfunction.

The answer to this self-defeating anticipatory and performance anxiety cycle is *not* a return to the youthful pattern of automatic, autonomous erections and total sexual confidence. Once sensitized to sexual problems, you cannot pretend it didn't happen and resume automatic functioning. After the first sexual failure, males have mixed experiences. By the time they seek therapy, the anxiety/failure pattern has become well-established. This results in secondary inhibited sexual desire. Sex is a source of anxiety, frustration and angst rather than pleasure.

Sexual anxiety and avoidance is stigmatizing because sex is seen as a measure of masculinity. The performance myth is "a real man can have sex with any woman, any time, any place." Yet you and your penis are human, not a perfect performance machine. How can you challenge this trap? Key concepts are positive, realistic sexual expectations, viewing your spouse as your intimate friend, enjoying nondemand pleasuring, allow pleasuring to flow into erotic stimulation, enjoying your own and the partner's arousal, viewing intercourse as a special erotic experience, letting arousal naturally flow to orgasm, enjoying afterplay. At its essence sexuality is about intimacy and pleasure not demands and performance. Desire and satisfaction are more important than arousal and orgasm. You are more than your penis, intercourse and ejaculation. Valuing intimate, interactive sex is a central concept. Sexuality is about sharing pleasure. Males have been socialized to function in a sexually autonomous manner, and only turn to the spouse when there is a problem. Openness to the spouse's stimulation and arousal is key to preventing dysfunction.

These strategies are particularly valuable for inhibited sexual desire, erectile dysfunction, and ejaculatory inhibition, but less so for the most common male problem, early ejaculation.

EARLY EJACULATION

The majority of males begin their sexual lives as early ejaculators. As they gain comfort and experience, most men develop ejaculatory control. However, three in ten adult males have a chronic problem of early ejaculation. The average time for intercourse from intromission to ejaculation is two to seven minutes. The great majority of males ejaculate in less than ten minutes.

People define early ejaculation in terms of time (a minute after intromission), activity (fewer than twenty strokes), or whether the woman is orgasmic during intercourse (an extremely poor criterion because a significant number of women are orgasmic in nonintercourse sex, not during intercourse). A reasonable approach is, if the couple are making good use of nongenital and genital pleasuring, and the man's ejaculation is earlier than they wish and interferes with pleasure, it is worthwhile to improve ejaculatory control. Learning ejaculatory control will enhance sexual pleasure for both the man and the couple.

Tara and Juan

When a sex therapist encounters a couple whose major problem is lack of knowledge and awareness, he can almost guarantee a successful outcome. Tara and Juan were in their mid-twenties, married two years, and feeling desperate about their sexual life. They were a loving couple and wanted sex to work in their marriage. Each time they had intercourse, Juan would ejaculate right at or shortly after intromission. Tara was neither aroused nor orgasmic. Juan was so discouraged that he avoided sex. They viewed the problem as Tara's not having an orgasm with the cause being Juan's early ejaculation.

After an assessment involving a couple session and individual sexual histories, the therapist reconceptualized the problem as two separate issues: Tara's arousal dysfunction and Juan's early ejaculation. Tara was not aroused before beginning intercourse. Juan was so concerned with early ejaculation that he avoided Tara's touch. Juan was bewildered, but willing, when the therapist suggested he spend time pleasuring Tara and be open to Tara's stimulating him.

The first step is being receptive to sensual, nongenital touch. Like many young men with early ejaculation, Juan's touch was rapid, rough, focused on her genitals, and goal-oriented. He needed to learn to touch in a slow, nondemanding, pleasure-oriented manner. He was surprised and pleased with Tara's responsiveness. Juan's openness to Tara's touch increased her arousal. Juan was not comfortable lying back and being passive, but he did enjoy being stimulated while he caressed her. Juan's rapid, goal-oriented sexual scenario had dampened her arousal. Slowing down the sexual scenario increased Tara's pleasure and arousal. As Juan became comfortable receiving genital stimulation, his ejaculatory control gradually increased. The key to learning ejaculatory control is building comfort, not reducing arousal. Tara found, as is true of many women, that if she was aroused and/or orgasmic during the pleasuring phase, it was easier to be aroused and orgasmic with intercourse.

Early ejaculation is a primary dysfunction, although some men (especially when sex is infrequent or tension-filled) develop secondary early ejaculation. The two most common male strategies make the problem worse. The first is "do it yourself" techniques to reduce arousal. These include biting your lip, wearing two condoms, thinking of the money you owe. The outcome of distraction techniques is reduced arousal, not ejaculatory control. You risk creating an erectile dysfunction. The second strategy is to replace quantity for quality, i.e., have a second intercourse as quickly as possible. Second orgasms are less satisfying for the man. The woman is more likely to feel like a sex object than a loved spouse. This negatively impacts couple sexuality—desire decreases because of low satisfaction.

Learning ejaculatory control is a three-phase process. First, identify the point of ejaculatory inevitability, after which ejaculation is no longer voluntary. Second, use the stop-start technique as you approach the point of inevitability. This enhances comfort, maintains arousal, and decreases anxiety. This is practiced utilizing manual stimulation and involves communicating to the spouse when to stop stimulation. The third phase involves ejaculatory control with intercourse. The couple practices intercourse in the female-on-top position using slow, long stroking (controlled by the woman). She stops stroking as he approaches the point of inevitability. As control increases, stroking is slowed rather than stopped. The couple experiment with intercourse positions, types of stroking, and rhythm of stroking. The hardest situation for ejaculatory control is with man on top with short, rapid thrusting.

Learning ejaculatory control is a couple task, requiring time, practice, and feedback. Ejaculatory control is not about the man performing to a standard or proving he can ''give'' the partner an orgasm during intercourse.

A common mistake is for sex to end at the man's ejaculation. Many women enjoy manual or rubbing stimulation after intercourse—either for orgasm or to share closeness. Afterplay is the most neglected phase of sexuality. Afterplay which emphasizes pleasure and bonding enhances the couple's (especially the woman's) satisfaction.

Learning ejaculatory control is like learning any skill. It is a gradual process requiring practice, feedback and working as an intimate team.

Doug and Alicia

Doug and Alicia fell into the traditional trap where he wanted to ignore or minimize the ejaculatory control problem and she wanted to cure it for him. When this didn't happen, Alicia became angry and Doug's worst critic.

Doug married Alicia at twenty-seven, joking that he finally got caught. In reality, he was glad to be married and looked forward to marital intimacy and security. Although he'd had sex with over twenty women, he'd never discussed the problem of early ejaculation. Doug focused on sexual quantity rather than quality, lasting longer the second time. Alicia had not raised the issue of early ejaculation. She had had fewer premarital partners, but the relationships had lasted longer. Often her partners gained ejaculatory control within six months. She'd naively hoped this would happen with Doug.

The "magic of romantic love sex" lasted eight months, ending six months before marriage. Doug and Alicia admit the quality of their premarital sex was mediocre, but fondly remember it as a very special time.

Romantic love fades even among the most intimate, sexually functional couples. Unless replaced by mature intimacy, the sexual relationship is vulnerable. Three months before marriage, Doug threatened to call it off because Alicia was saying no to sex with increasing frequency. Rather than dealing with issues of sexual desire and early ejaculation, Alicia placated Doug. This proved disastrous for both. Alicia felt sexually anxious and pressured. Increasingly she resented Doug, feeling alienated and less aroused. Alicia's desire, involvement, and orgasms decreased. Doug felt it was on his shoulders to maintain sex, and his focus was quantity.

A year and a half into the marriage, the problem of early ejaculation was raised, this time with more vehemence and less empathy. After a frustrating experience, Alicia blew up and accused Doug of being uncaring and sexually selfish. He was shocked, offended, and counterattacked by calling her a "frigid bitch." Alicia saw him as cruel and withdrew. Impulsive sexual fights in bed are volatile and counterproductive.

Doug decided he'd show her by achieving ejaculatory control on his own. He used as his resource an advertisement in a men's magazine offering a desensitizing cream with a money back guarantee. All it did was irritate his penis. Doug consulted a male sex clinic, which prescribed a low dose of antidepressant medication (Prozac, the new miracle drug). He didn't tell Alicia about this, but was pleased ejaculatory control improved. When Alicia found the medication, she was very concerned about Doug's depression. He felt embarrassed and threw out the pills. Early ejaculation returned with a vengeance. Medication can help establish ejaculatory control, but is not a miracle cure. If incorporated into a couple's ejaculatory control program, medication can be a valuable resource. However, if done alone, especially kept secret from the spouse, it's likely to backfire and cause alienation.

Doug's strategy had been to do it himself to prove something to Alicia. Unfortunately, he wound up with a worse problem—erectile anxiety. He inserted as soon as he became erect, ejaculated at or right after intromission, and blamed it on Alicia's sexual disinterest. This demonstrates the iatrogenic effect of focusing on sexual performance—it creates a more severe sexual problem. It wasn't long before Doug and Alicia were avoiding not only intercourse but affectionate touch. They were stuck in the cycle of emotional alienation, inhibited desire, and avoidance.

It was Alicia who suggested couples sex therapy. Alicia had been in individual therapy as a college student and two years of group therapy as an adult. Doug was distrustful of psychotherapy, but open to the idea of sex therapy. Regaining comfort and confidence with erection was the first focus. Doug approached Alicia as an intimate friend and shared sexual concerns and anxieties, as well as sexual requests and turn-ons. Alicia was a willing and supportive spouse. The initial exercises involving pleasuring made Alicia feel very good, and her enthusiasm transferred to Doug. This is the pattern—women find sex therapy concepts and techniques easier to accept than men. Intimacy and nondemand pleasuring greatly enhanced Alicia's sexual anticipation and desire. Her openness and desire increased Doug's involvement and arousal. With manual and oral stimulation, Doug was surprised how quickly his erectile confidence returned. Sex was no longer a race toward erection, intercourse, and ejaculation. Slowing down the process while increasing erotic stimulation resulted in better erections and ejaculatory control.

A breakthrough occurred when they began using the stop-start technique. Alicia did manual and oral stimulation, and when Doug approached the point of ejaculatory inevitability he signaled her to stop. They did this for eight to twelve minutes, communicating feelings and enjoying eroticism. Although Alicia found it less fun after the first week, both knew they could master ejaculatory control if they worked together. Being intimate friends where each spouse's arousal enhances the other's was particularly valuable. Doug wasn't performing for Alicia, they were sharing pleasure and eroticism.

In the transition to intercourse, Alicia guided intromission. She began with slow, long thrusting. They used the stop-start technique before and during intercourse. What worked even better was changing the type and rhythm of coital thrusting. Alicia was orgasmic with both intercourse and nonintercourse stimulation. Doug was learning ejaculatory control not for Alicia to have an orgasm during intercourse (although he did enjoy this), but to make the sexual experience comfortable, pleasurable, erotic, and satisfying for both of them.

ERECTILE DYSFUNCTION

Far too much of a man's self-esteem is tied to his penis. Erectile dysfunction (commonly called "impotence" or "not getting it up") is a major male fear. A well-hidden fact is that by age forty, ninety percent of men have experienced (at least once) a problem with obtaining or maintaining an erection adequate for intercourse. By age fifty, one in three males reports erectile difficulty. So the man's major fear is, in fact, an almost universal experience. Men are notorious liars and braggarts about sexual prowess. They deny sexual doubts, questions, or difficulties. The myth-based performance criterion of "a real man is able and willing to have sex with any woman, at any time, in any situation" puts tremendous pressure on him—and his penis.

For men under fifty, the great majority of erectile problems are caused by psychological or relationship problems rather than physical or medical factors. Physical vulnerabilities increase with age. Common physical causes include alcohol abuse, side effects of medications (especially hypertension and psychiatric medications), spinal injury, prostate surgery, chronic illness, poorly controlled diabetes, and vascular insufficiency. Common psychological and relational causes are anticipatory anxiety, performance anxiety, distraction, viewing intercourse as a pass-fail test, work or parenting stress, reluctance to be dependent on partner stimulation, and anger at the spouse. If an erection problem does not remit within six months, the man (and couple) become trapped in the cycle of anticipatory anxiety, performance failure, and avoidance. No matter what started the problem (alcohol, side effect of medication, fatigue, alienation, depression, anger, trying to force sex), this cycle maintains erectile dysfunction.

The hormonal, vascular, and neurological systems must be functional for erectile response. With aging, beginning in one's mid-thirties, there is a gradual decline in the efficacy of these systems. That's why there are few professional athletes at age forty—the body is a less efficient performance machine. Lowered testosterone affects sexual desire, which indirectly effects erectile functioning. An erection involves increased blood flow to the penis (vasocongestion), which fills the tissues and increases size. As arousal builds, rigidity (hardness) increases—a neurological response. These systems remain functional, but no longer at optimal efficiency. Psychological, relational and erotic factors become crucial for erectile response.

Erection is vulnerable to distraction and anxiety. Intimacy, nondemand pleasuring, and erotic stimulation become more important in promoting erectile comfort and confidence. A fifty-year-old man is not the easy, automatic, autonomous sexual machine he was at twenty. Sexual response is more variable. Both spouses can accept sexual variability and flexibility while maintaining positive sexual feelings and expectations.

If you have questions about physical or medical aspects of sexual functioning, the doctor to consult is a urologist. Although not considered a male sex doctor, the urologist functions much the way a gynecologist does for women. Be sure the urologist is interested in doing a comprehensive assessment, not simply promoting prosthesis surgery, penile injections, external pumps, or oral medications.

The most important assessment question is whether the man is able to get erections during self-stimulation, with manual or oral stimulation, during sleep, or on awakening. If so, it's likely that physical components are functional, although operating at less efficiency, especially after age fifty. Anxiety, distraction, fatigue, negative emotions are major factors interfering with sexual functioning. Psychological factors of comfort, involvement, intimacy and openness are necessary to regain erectile confidence. These include communication with and trust of the spouse, being turned on by her arousal and open to her stimulation, making sexual requests. Erotic factors, especially penile stimulation, her guiding intromission, awareness of personal and couple turn-ons, and enjoying nonintercourse sex to orgasm are crucial. If the couple chooses to use medical aides such as an injection, oral medication, or external pump, they have to communicate and integrate these into their lovemaking style.

Guidelines for change emphasize intimacy, nondemand pleasuring, erotic stimulation, and positive, realistic expectations. As with other sexual problems, seeking the counsel of a sex therapist is superior to working on your own. The foundation is nongenital and genital pleasuring, giving and receiving pleasure-oriented touch with a temporary prohibition on intercourse. A crucial technique is the man and woman becoming comfortable with the waxing and waning of erections. The man is used to going to intercourse and orgasm on a first erection, so when the erection fades he panics. He's afraid the sexual opportunity is lost. Continued involvement and erotic stimulation ensures the erection will wax (gain strength) again. This process can occur two to five times in a forty-five-minute pleasuring session. The next step is to be orgasmic at least twice while erect during nonintercourse sex (manual, oral, or rubbing stimulation). This increases awareness of the interplay between subjective and objective arousal. With continual, free flow of penile stimulation he is orgasmic. Subjective arousal (feeling turned on) usually proceeds to objective arousal (becoming erect). Without the fear of intercourse failure, arousal and orgasm flow. The next step is to play with the penis around the vagina to desensitize performance anxiety and give the woman practice at stimulating and guiding the penis. She decides when to transition to intercourse, what position to use, and guides intromission. During intercourse, the couple is encouraged to use multiple stimulation (he touching her breasts, she stroking his testicles, kissing, doing clitoral stimulation, fantasizing) which builds erotic feelings, heightens arousal, and flows to orgasm.

Men who overcome erectile dysfunction don't go back to easy, automatic erections. They are aware lovers who have comfort and confidence with erections and appreciate variable, flexible sexual expression. Approximately 85 percent of sexual experiences flow into intercourse, another 5-10 percent involve non-intercourse sex. Mediocre or disappointing sexual experiences (5-10 percent) are accepted. If sex gets off track, it's seen as a lapse, not a relapse. Men (and couples) who can shrug off or laugh about disappointing or unsuccessful sexual experiences are in a solid position to maintain erectile comfort and confidence.

Sarah and Sam

Often the roadblock to sexual arousal involves a relationship problem. Sarah and Sam met while married to other people. Sarah married seven years ago because of a pregnancy; the husband wanted them to stay together for the daughter's sake. Sarah realized they were better as parents than spouses or lovers (they hadn't been sexual in three years). Sarah's parents had stayed together "for the sake of the children." She did not want to repeat that pattern in her life.

Sarah saw the relationship with Sam as a transition to being single again. She was attracted to Sam and enamored by his attention and passionate wooing of her. Ten weeks after meeting Sam, Sarah left her husband. Up to that point sex with Sam had been excellent. They met at hotels for "nooners" and went away for a weekend. Sarah remembers it as the most sexually free time of her life.

During his marriage, Sam had adopted a pattern of affairs that lasted from two weeks to two years. After eight years of marriage, he had erection problems with his wife. Although they occasionally had intercourse, he never regained erectile confidence in marital sex. Erections were easy early in an affair, so he told himself arousal problems reflected the fact that he was a man who required new partners. Sam preached "Man is not meant to be monogamous." When erection problems began, he immediately dropped the relationship.

Sarah told Sam the coming months were likely to be a "crazy time." The first priority was to get her life back to an equilibrium and set up a coparenting arrangement. Their relationship would not be as much fun, so she would understand if he ended it. Sam

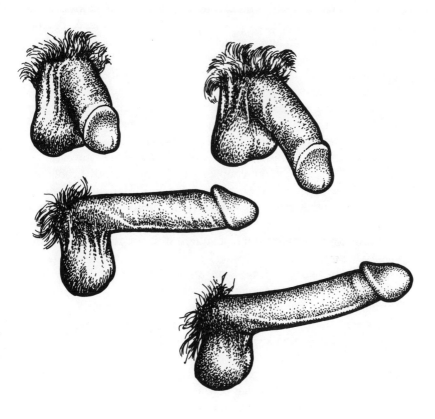

Erections can and do wax and wane. Understanding and accepting that process is key to regaining erectile confidence.

surprised himself by staying. He rationalized that even if sex wasn't as frequent, it was still passionate and fulfilling. Sarah's arousal remained high—sex with Sam was a tension-reducer and energized her to cope with problems. She was finding it difficult to convince her exspouse to stop fighting to get her back and accept the inevitability of divorce.

Sam's first problem with erection occurred four months after Sarah's separation. He was sure Sarah hadn't noticed, but he rushed intromission and ejaculation so there wouldn't be an erectile "failure." Sam was sensitized and self-conscious about erection, and began avoiding sex. Two months later, they were being sexual at Sarah's initiation, and Sam lost his erection before intromission. Sarah was a sexually aware and sophisticated woman who knew this occasionally happened and didn't make an issue of it. Sam felt humiliated, turned against Sarah, and blamed her aggressiveness. Sarah felt unjustly attacked and they got into the kind of destructive fight couples have about sexual problems. Sarah fully expected Sam to terminate the relationship, which was Sam's intent in provoking the fight. He found to his amazement that he couldn't do it. Sam loved and respected Sarah, and couldn't walk away from the healthiest intimate relationship he'd ever had.

The next two years were an emotional roller coaster. Sam separated from his wife. Sarah agreed to live with Sam to determine if they were a viable couple. Could Sarah and Sam sustain their commitment and establish an intimate, secure second marriage? Sarah realized anger and feeling emotionally distant squelched sexual desire. When she was receptive to touching, she had little difficulty becoming aroused. Sam understood that the exact same sexual scenario which resulted in passionate feelings and multiorgasmic response when Sarah was open resulted in dead feelings when she was not receptive.

Sarah did not take Sam's erectile difficulties personally nor did she view erection as a sign of love or her sexual attractiveness. She correctly labeled the erectile difficulty a "psychological block." Too much of a man's self-esteem lies in his penis. This was certainly true for Sam. The key to regaining sexual comfort and confidence is viewing the partner as your sexual friend, seeing sexuality as pleasure-giving and pleasure-receiving rather than a pass-fail performance, and viewing intercourse as part of the pleasuring process. Sam heard these concepts in therapy sessions, read them in sexuality books, and experienced with Sarah the waxing and waning of erections. Sarah stimulated him manually and orally, and guided his penis into her. As is true of many males, Sam was stubborn when it came to changing sexual attitudes and behavior. He felt that without a guarantee of a strong erection, sex would never feel right. The emotional breakthrough came one morning when he awoke with an erection. He tried to initiate a quick intercourse, but lost his erection. Rather than allow him to slip into a feeling-sorry-for-himself mood, Sarah asked to cuddle. She was responsive to his touch. When he began to stimulate her toward orgasm, she moved his hand from her genitals to her chest and said she just wanted to feel close. He did not worry about his penis, but stayed with feelings of pleasure. In the next twenty minutes his erection waxed and waned two or three times, but he did not become distracted. When Sarah got on top and guided him into her it seemed the most natural thing possible. After that, sex between Sarah and Sam went smoothly with no major roadblocks. On those occasions when his erection was not firm, they felt free to engage in alternate sensual or erotic scenarios.

EJACULATORY INHIBITION

This is the least known male sexual dysfunction. The old terms "retarded ejaculation" or "ejaculatory incompetence" had a negative, put-down connotation. Ejaculatory inhibition refers to the man wanting to reach orgasm, but his sexual response is blocked (inhibited). The most severe form, primary ejaculatory inhibition (inability to ejaculate by any means), is extremely rare. Among young men the most common manifestation is the inability to ejaculate during intercourse, although he does with masturbation (and usually with manual or oral stimulation). This can continue for years, not being addressed until the couple wants to become pregnant.

Ejaculatory inhibition is most common in the intermittent form, affecting as many as fifteen percent of men, especially after age fifty. Inability or difficulty ejaculating stems from a range of inhibitions—inability to let go, beginning intercourse at low levels of arousal, lack of comfort requesting erotic stimulation, fear or ambivalence about pregnancy, feeling sexually guilty or fearful. Some males reach orgasm with a very narrow type of stimulation—rubbing against bedsheets, a fetish arousal pattern, self-stimulation with partner present—but are inhibited during interactive sex. Sex is a cooperative, sharing experience between two people who are involved in giving and receiving pleasure. With ejaculatory inhibition, this process is blocked. Rather than orgasm being the natural culmination of arousal, it becomes an anxiety-provoking goal he fails to achieve.

As with other sexual dysfunctions, ejaculatory inhibition is best seen as a couple issue. The couple—not just the man—increases involvement and eroticism. You cannot will or force an orgasm—the key is increased arousal, especially subjective feelings of being turned on. Erections (objective arousal) can occur at low levels of subjective arousal, so she mistakenly believes he's highly aroused. A typical inhibition is feeling shy about requesting erotic scenarios and stimulation.

Two techniques to facilitate orgasm are multiple stimulation and orgasm triggers. Men with ejaculatory inhibition have intercourse for half an hour, an hour, or longer. Males suffering from early ejaculation or worrying about erections envy these men. What nonsense. Intercourse is mechanical (and sometimes aversive), not pleasurable. Involvement and arousal remain static. Intercourse is to service the partner rather than give and get pleasure. A guideline is not to initiate intercourse until subjective arousal is at least a "5" and preferably a "7" on a 10-point scale of arousal. Another is to request erotic stimulation—which can involve fellatio while he moves rhythmically, stroking buttocks or testicles, combining kissing and manual stimulation. Continue erotic stimulation during intercourse. Why should multiple stimulation cease when intercourse begins? Erotic stimulation involves giving as well as receiving stimulation. You can switch intercourse positions. She does testicle or chest stimulation while he gives breast or clitoral stimulation. He can verbalize erotic feelings, fantasize or tell erotic stories.

Orgasm triggers are idiosyncratic. One of the best ways to identify orgasm triggers is to tune into the touches, thoughts, fantasies, and movements you utilize right before the point of ejaculatory inevitability during masturbation. Transfer these to partner sex. Orgasm triggers include verbalizing or making sounds, moving your body, focusing on a fantasy, giving stimulation, watching the partner, doing rhythmic thrusting. Orgasm triggers allow you to transition from high arousal to letting go and coming.

Jack and Trudi

Intermittent ejaculatory inhibition often increases in the middle years. As many as fifteen percent of men experience this. Jack was an early ejaculator in his mid-twenties; it was not until his mid-thirties that he developed ejaculatory control. He became comfortable with and open to Trudi's stimulation. Their intercourse frequency was two or three times a week (a regular rhythm of intercourse promotes ejaculatory control). Trudi did not begin having orgasms until two years into the marriage, and by her mid-thirties was orgasmic two thirds of the time. Her favorite sexual scenario was to begin with kissing and caressing, which facilitated openness to Jack's stimulation. Trudi especially enjoyed receiving a sexual massage. As arousal built, Trudi moved toward orgasm by thrusting her pelvis while Jack stimulated her with his penis, hand, or tongue. Jack enjoyed her arousal, which added to his.

Throughout this book we have made the point that you cannot rest on your laurels. This is the trap Trudi and Jack fell into. By their late forties, Jack felt sex was easier and better for Trudi. Jack didn't voice his feelings, which festered and grew more invasive. It is normal for a male occasionally not to reach orgasm, the major reason being that arousal is moderate and remains so throughout intercourse. The male is considered to have ejaculatory inhibition when during at least one in four opportunities he is aroused and desirous of having a climax but unable to. Over the previous five years the occurrences of ejaculatory inhibition increased, but neither Jack nor Trudi addressed the problem. Orgasm does not exist in a vacuum. Trudi's arousal also began to decline. Their sexual relationship was on a downhill slope, and the next stop was inhibited sexual desire.

Trudi took the initiative to break the cycle. She bought *Male Sexual Awareness* and underlined three concepts she thought were relevant—multiple stimulation, requests for special sexual scenarios, and using orgasm triggers. She left this under Jacks's

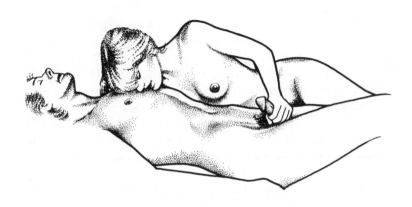

The spouse is your intimate friend—be open to her touch and stimulation.

pillow with a cute note about winning a sexual prize. She bought a pair of sexy short pajamas that provided a nice touch.

What turned things around was a sexual scenario in which Trudi brought Jack to orgasm orally, something they hadn't done in five years. The next morning she told Jack she enjoyed helping him get excited and have an orgasm, it was arousing for her when he was aroused. Jack acknowledged how nice it had been and how free he felt. Jack shared a story about how a work colleague, who had been frustrated and resentful toward his wife, acted out by having an affair with a divorced, younger secretary, and how this disrupted the work environment and marriage. Jack told Trudi he valued their life and marriage, but admitted he'd been frustrated with sex. He didn't expect miracle changes, but last night had been a great start.

Jack read the book and identified the problem: as Trudi became more aroused she'd stop stimulating him, and his arousal waned. He didn't say anything because he didn't want to be a crybaby. Jack needed Trudi's continued stimulation for arousal to build to orgasm. They agreed to experiment and play together to develop erotic scenarios. Middle-years sex is not as easy and predictable as youthful sex. If the man can make sexual requests and enjoy give-and-take stimulation, middle-years sex can be high-quality and satisfying. An involved, aroused partner is the major aphrodisiac.

SEXUAL VARIATIONS

Approximately two to five percent of males have a variant arousal pattern. The most common types are fetish arousal, cross-dressing, 900 numbers with a specialty in "kinky" fantasies, cybersex, and sadomasochistic behavior. A second category is a "noxious paraphilia," a sexual arousal pattern which is abusive and illegal. This includes exhibitionism, voyeurism, obscene phone calls, and pedophilia.

Variant arousal is very narrow, but very powerful. It's quite difficult, and usually impossible, to transfer to couple sex. Premaritally and early in the marriage the man might be functional, but over time he develops inhibited sexual desire. Desire for intimate, interactive sex is low. Sexual desire is trapped in the narrow dead-end of variant arousal.

Let's consider the more serious problem first, noxious para-philia. This behavior is illegal and harmful to others. The pattern develops in childhood or early adolescence and is reinforced by thousands of experiences masturbating to images of deviant arousal. It's best thought of as a compulsive, addictive behavior which serves as the man's "secret sexual world." He distorts reality by pretending it's OK and does no harm. Couple sex can't compete with this distorted fantasy and secret world.

This problem absolutely requires clinical intervention. The man is in denial or minimizes the impact of the deviant arousal. He is intent on keeping this secret from the spouse. The secret is exposed when he's arrested—a major crisis for the man and the marriage. Prevention is preferable to crisis management. This problem will not be resolved unless addressed therapeutically.

Fetishism, cross-dressing, masturbating to pornography, tele-phone or on-line sex, going to prostitutes or massage parlors, doesn't involve illegal activity or harm others. However, it's very impactful, subverting couple intimacy. The woman feels relieved when the problem is revealed, because she blamed herself or felt "crazy." Rather than feeling involved and turned on during part-ner sex, he tries to shut her off and focus on fantasies. Most men, and many women, use fantasies as a bridge to arousal, a healthy form of erotic stimulation. However, variant fantasies serve as a wall to block out the partner. Intimacy is a victim of variant arousal.

The therapeutic strategy is a one two combination of the male confronting and breaking the variant arousal pattern and the cou-ple developing an intimate, interactive sexual style. The woman is not responsible for changing the man's variant arousal, he is. It's a joint responsibility to develop a comfortable, functional couple sexual style.

CLOSING THOUGHTS

Male sexual dysfunction usually precedes inhibited sexual de-sire. The man is embarrassed and humiliated because he cannot meet the rigid performance demands he grew up with. He retreats into blaming himself, blaming the spouse, and sexual avoidance. The key to change is to adopt a broad, flexible, pleasure-oriented approach to sexuality. The couple is an intimate team that develops a comfortable, functional sexual style. Couples sex therapy facilitates this process. Trying to change on his own is likely to be iatrogenic and cause more serious marital and sexual problems. The key to change is regaining sexual comfort and confidence and viewing the spouse as your intimate friend.

15

PARTNERS IN HEALING—DEALING WITH SEXUAL TRAUMA

Sexual trauma isn't supposed to happen to married adults. Yet, the reality is that perhaps thirty percent of couples have to deal with past or present sexual trauma. Sometimes this involves dealing with childhood experiences, sometimes experiences which occur during the marriage, and sometimes sexual trauma occurring with one's children.

Sexual trauma is a complex, sensitive, and controversial area which has a multitude of causes, dimensions and outcomes. We focus on two themes:

1. Negative or traumatic sexual experiences occur in childhood, adolescence, and adulthood. These must be dealt with rather than denied and treated as a shameful secret at one extreme or allowed to be the controlling factor governing your sexuality and marriage on the other extreme. A core cognition is thinking of yourself as a "survivor," not a "victim." A second core cognition is "living well is the best revenge."

2. Dealing with sexual trauma is a couple issue, not just the burden of the person who's been traumatized. The traumatic incident affects not only the individual, but the spouse and their intimate relationship. The spouse is a "partner in healing." You need to be there emotionally, talking about and dealing with the incident rather than becoming trapped in guilt or blame. Integrate the traumatic experience in a way which accepts and honors the feelings connected to it, but does not allow them to dominate your self-esteem, sexuality or intimate relationship. Being a sur-

vivor allows you to regain control of your body and touch. You value pleasure-oriented, voluntary, intimate sexuality. Dealing with sexual trauma cannot be achieved through reading a book, attending a lecture, watching a TV program, or listening to a talk show. This increases awareness and understanding, but is not enough. Resolving sexual trauma requires professional therapy. In this chapter we hope to increase awareness and suggest guidelines for addressing issues.

TYPES OF SEXUAL TRAUMA

Sexual trauma is more than the "big three" of child sexual abuse, incest, and rape. If you define negative sexual experiences broadly—to include contracting a sexually transmitted disease, being sexually humiliated, having an unwanted pregnancy, guilt over masturbation, being exhibited to or peeped on, receiving obscene phone calls, being sexually harassed, having a sexual dysfunction, a compulsive sexual pattern, being sexually rejected—you are confronted with a disturbing realization. Negative, confusing, abusive or traumatic sexual experiences are an almost universal phenomenon for men as well as women. Over ninety percent of women and men identify at least one sexual incident (whether in childhood, adolescence, or adulthood) that caused negative feelings or trauma.

Stigma and sense of victimization is more psychologically traumatic than the sexual incident itself. There are three levels of victimization: (1) the sexual incident; (2) how the incident was dealt with at the time; (3) the long-term effect—does she see herself (sexual self-esteem) as a "survivor" or a "victim"? For example, a nine-year-old girl is sexually abused by a male neighbor, brother-in-law, or teacher (over ninety percent of perpetrators are male, whether the child is male or female). The most common age for abuse is between eight and twelve. The most common activity is touching the girl's breasts or vulva. That is the first level of abuse—the sexual incident. The second level is how the incident is dealt with at the time—does she keep it secret (resulting in a sense of shame or depression) or does she tell someone (a parent, teacher, friend's mother). Although telling someone is healthy, often the result for the child is more confusion, anxiety and stigma. Her feelings and needs weren't listened to. The third level is how the person has integrated the incident into her adult self-esteem. Too often, she feels like a victim, whether a passive, shameful victim or an angry, acting-out victim. Ideally, she would see herself as a proud survivor who coped as well as she could at the time. As an adult she feels she deserves a mutual, voluntary, pleasure-oriented and intimate sexual life.

Approximately one in three female children and one in seven male children by age fourteen have a sexual incident with an adult or adolescent (at least five years older). This might be hands-on abuse—touching the child's genitals or buttocks, or coercing the child to touch the adult's genitals. Half of the incidents with female children involve hands-off abuse (voyeurism, exhibitionism, sexual harassment, obscene phone calls or viewing pornography). Most abuse of boys is hands-on and usually involves orgasm-related activity (fellating the boy to orgasm, having the boy manually or orally stimulate the man to orgasm, being passive in anal intercourse). Traditionally, children told no one, they felt the abuse was their fault, it was a shameful secret. If the child did tell a family member or teacher, the tendency was not to believe her, deny or minimize the incident, and/or be angry at the child. Traditionally, our culture "blames the victim." This tendency is at its worst in sexual abuse of boys.

Most abuse is nonintercourse, nonviolent, and involves someone the child knows. This is contrary to the cultural stereotype, that the perpetrator is a stranger who forces intercourse. Factors which increase trauma include use of force, ongoing secrets, a family member or trusted authority figure (minister, teacher, counselor, youth leader), and the child being manipulated to feel responsible for the abuse.

Incest is traumatic because it violates a trust bond. Incest is harmful both psychologically and sexually. The most frequent forms of incestuous behavior involve cousins, in-laws, siblings, and uncles. Most incidents involve viewing, fondling, manual or oral stimulation. Most involve female children, but male children are victimized more than people realize. The relationship which has the most negative impact is between a father and daughter or son. What allows incest to continue is silence, secrecy, and shame. Incest is an example of the man's deviant sexual desire causing harm to children, himself, and the entire family. Incest must not remain a shameful family secret. It needs to be confronted, dealt with, and stopped.

The majority of rape incidents involve someone the woman knows rather than a stranger. Rape is the double standard taken to its illogical extreme. Rape is legally defined as penis-vagina intercourse, but any forced or coerced sexual act is rape, including oral sex, anal intercourse, or manual sex. Rape is an act of violence, not just a sexual act. However, being raped is different than being mugged. The combination of violence and sexuality makes rape a particularly traumatic experience. For most middle-class women, rape is their first experience with violence. Two thirds of women report psychological distress three months after the rape. Rape not only affects the woman, but significant people in her life including spouse, family, and friends. They are co-victims, feeling the stress and being unsure how they feel or how to react to her.

DEALING WITH A HISTORY OF CHILD SEXUAL ABUSE OR INCEST

When one spouse has a history of child sexual abuse or incest, the psychologically healthy response is to share that with the partner. Sharing vulnerabilities and secrets promotes self-esteem and builds the trust bond. A favorite adage is, "You're only as sick as your secrets." Unfortunately, less than one in five people follows this guideline. Whether the secret is having an abortion or a child placed for adoption, a sexually transmitted disease or guilt over a destructive affair, child sexual abuse or incest, it is not disclosed. The dating/mating ritual is to present oneself in the most positive light and avoid revealing problems or vulnerabilities. This results in conflict later when the spouse feels tricked or manipulated or asks, Why didn't you tell me.

In sharing sexually sensitive issues from childhood or adolescence, make the spouse aware of your vulnerabilities and "traps" so she can be your emotional and sexual ally. This helps prevent problems with intimacy or sexual problems. Psychologically, prevention is the optimal strategy. Failing that, mobilize yourselves to understand and deal with the problem in its acute phase when you feel like an intimate team dealing with a common enemy. If the problem is chronic and you are in a guilt-blame cycle, it's time to seek therapy. Layers of frustration, resentment, self-blame and blame of the spouse compound the problem. One of the most powerful therapeutic interventions is helping the person to disclose her painful sexual secret and enlist the spouse as a partner in healing. Much of the turmoil could have been prevented if the spouse had discussed the sexual abuse and traps to be aware of. Unfortunately, intimacy is easily subverted, especially by sexual secrets.

Rosa and Alberto

Rosa and Alberto had a vibrant sexual relationship before marriage. After she became pregnant in the second month of marriage, sex abruptly stopped. Initially, they blamed it on morning sickness and then on sleep deprivation during the first two years of their daughter's life. Alberto felt trapped in a nonsexual marriage. His resentment and blaming of Rosa was intense. Rosa felt coerced and appalled by Roberto's behavior. She didn't want to have sex with a man she didn't trust and who abused her. The sexual power struggle threatened to result in divorce.

At the suggestion of their minister, Rosa and Alberto consulted a marriage therapist with a reputation for saving marriages. The therapy focus was on intimacy and sexual issues. In the individual history session, she asked Rosa about the most confusing, guilt-inducing, or traumatic sexual experience during the eighteen years she had lived at home. The therapist was the first person Rosa told about the sexual abuse when she was nine years old with a cousin who was eight years older. Since it did not involve intercourse, Rosa hadn't labeled this sexual abuse. The cousin had Rosa fellate him to orgasm, he stimulated her breasts and vulva, and spanked her. Rosa felt guilt and shame because she found it exciting. So how could this be abuse? The essence of childhood sexual abuse is that the man's sexual needs override the child's emotional needs. Child sexual abuse and incest is psychologically and sexually harmful. It can subvert the person's sexual desire and functioning in adulthood. Rosa was an excellent example.

When sex was new, illicit, and adventuresome, Rosa was desirous and responsive. However, when the relationship required trust and integration of intimacy and sexuality, Rosa found it extremely difficult. When Alberto became frustrated and verbally attacked her, Rosa became defensive and counterattacked. Misunderstanding, frustration, and resentment built. Although they worked together on parenting, they were emotionally alienated. It wasn't just sexual intercourse that stopped, but affectionate touching and sensuality ceased. Rosa didn't trust Alberto, why should she trust him with her body or her sexual secret?

When they arrived for the couple feedback session, the tension in the room was palpable. When the therapist asked Alberto what he feared hearing, it was that Rosa was having an affair and would leave him for the other man. Rosa was shocked. An affair was the farthest thing from her mind. When asked about her fears concerning Alberto, Rosa said he no longer found her sexually attractive and would abandon her and their child. Alberto's reaction was anger, he was not the kind of man who would leave his wife and family. The therapist helped them confront the guilt-blame trap, and increase understanding and empathy for each other's hurt and pain.

Disclosing Rosa's history of incest had a dramatic impact. Rosa was afraid she'd be blamed for all sexual problems and seen as "spoiled goods." Roberto was shocked to hear what had happened and cried for her pain, both as a child and having to keep this secret. Roberto's empathy and concern was genuine. For the first time in three years, Rosa thought of him as her intimate spouse and supporter. Empathy was the crucial missing ingredient. With increased trust and empathy, the power struggle began to melt.

Rosa and Alberto needed to confront the reality of the sexual abuse history and establish a voluntary, mutual, pleasure-oriented, and communicative relationship. Sexual trauma and inhibited sexual desire were a common enemy, which needed to be addressed by both as an intimate team. A key agreement was that Alberto would honor Rosa's veto of any sexual interaction which made her self-conscious or uncomfortable. Rosa committed to not avoid touching or intimacy. Therapy was slow and complex. The foundation for change was healing touch and intimacy. Rosa saw Alberto as her trusted, intimate spouse who valued her. They successfully integrated intimacy and sexuality into their marital bond.

RAPE AS A MARRIED ADULT

Marriage meets needs for intimacy and security better than any other relationship. Married women don't expect to be raped. However, marriage does not protect against rape, whether by a stranger or an acquaintance.

The rape of a spouse is a traumatic experience for both the woman and her husband, and a major stress on their marital bond. Although this is irrational, it is easier for the husband to be supportive if it was a rape by a stranger and or there was physical violence. This is not true for the woman. For many women, rape is their first experience with extreme violence. Fear of death, physical pain, being out of control of your body, is frightening. The combination of sex and violence makes rape particularly traumatic.

In a nonviolent (i.e., without weapons or bruises) acquaintance rape, it's easier for the woman to fall into the trap of blaming herself. Likewise, the husband falls into the trap of blaming the spouse and taking his frustration and anger out on her. He questions her judgment and calls her stupid for getting into a vulnerable situation. By blaming the spouse he is doubly victimizing her and harming their relationship. She needs acceptance and support, not criticism and put-downs.

To be a partner in healing, he needs to listen in a respectful, caring manner. Her feelings and needs come first in dealing with the crisis. In a rape, the perpetrator's needs are met at the woman's expense, sex is forced or coerced, her physical and emotional boundaries are violated. In helping her cope and be a survivor, the husband's role is that of her trusted, intimate friend. Her feelings and needs have priority. When she is uncomfortable or vetoes touch, even a hug, her rights and personal boundaries are respected. The couple proceeds at her pace, not his. Together, you regain comfort and confidence with intimacy and sexuality. Healing is more likely if you utilize the services of a therapist rather than proceeding on your own.

Touch—whether affectionate, sensual, or sexual—is voluntary, mutual, pleasure-oriented. Healing from rape focuses on "Living well is the best revenge." The rapist no longer controls her sexual self-esteem or their intimate bond. Rape is the opposite of intimacy. Regaining desire, arousal, orgasm, and satisfaction is integral to healing, but not the central factor. The core is for the victim to regain a sense of personal integrity, trust in herself and intimate relationship, feeling pride in being a survivor and the relationship with her partner having survived. A rape is an attack on the woman, with the husband a covictim. Being partners in healing is integral to regaining control of your body, sexuality, and intimate relationship.

Melissa and Charles

Neither Melissa nor Charles ever thought they'd have to deal with a rape incident, especially since Melissa was forty-one. However, at an office Christmas party a colleague got quite drunk. Melissa had three drinks, and although not drunk, her awareness and judgment were impaired. She did not see potential danger in his suggestive dancing, touching her, and sexual innuendos—instead, she mistakenly labeled it as playful and harmless flirtation. He was fifteen years younger, and Melissa found it cute that a younger man found her attractive. He walked her to her car and under the guise of concern for her well-being checked to be sure no one was hiding in the back seat. Melissa was shocked and confused when he pulled her into the back seat. As he ripped at her clothes she felt paralyzed, unable to react and abort this. When she did say stop and moved to extricate herself, he seemed in a frenzy of anger and lust. The whole incident couldn't have lasted more than ten minutes.

Melissa was terrified and totally disoriented. She got her clothes on and drove home. Melissa avoided Charles—all she wanted was to get out of her clothes, shower and go to sleep. However, she was too agitated to sleep. Melissa felt she had no one to talk to. Had this been a sexual assault? Was it her fault? Should she tell Charles? Would he blame her? How could she go to work and face this man? Should she file a complaint at work? Should she call the police? At four A.M., Melissa called the rape crisis hotline. She felt listened to and believed, but the suggestion to send a rape companion to her house and accompany her to the emergency room and police station was not the way Melissa wanted to proceed. This might be right for some women, but not for Melissa. At eight that morning, Melissa called her best friend, saying she needed to talk about a crisis and asked if she could come over for coffee. The friend was very supportive and helped Melissa talk through the incident and examine her feelings and alternatives. Melissa understood that this was a sexual assault (acquaintance rape). It was the perpetrator's responsibility, and she had no reason to feel guilty. She needed to share this with Charles and needed his understanding and support. In terms of the workplace, she valued her job and didn't want to feel on the defensive. The friend told Melissa she needed to sleep. Later, she would keep the children so Melissa and Charles would have the privacy to talk.

When Melissa awoke she called Charles to come home from work early. Charles came home with the expectation that Melissa was planning a sexual get-together, but when he saw her he knew something serious had happened. He was shocked to hear her story. Charles cried with her and held her. His initial reaction was to beat the man and then call the police, but realized this was not what Melissa wanted or needed. The ''super macho'' aggressive strategy was for Charles's needs, not Melissa's. Melissa wanted to be held, emotionally supported, not feel blamed, and to know Charles would be there for her. They decided not to share the incident with their nine and seven-year-old children, not out of shame, but because it would not be helpful for the family. Charles agreed to be the prime parent for the Christmas season. He also agreed to help Melissa draft a memo to the president of the company and chief of human resources detailing the sexual assault and request that the man be discharged from the company.

Charles agreed to follow Melissa's lead regarding their intimate relationship. She could veto any touch which was uncomfortable. Regaining trust and intimacy was not as easy or straightforward as either Charles or Melissa hoped. The healing process, regaining comfort with touch and regaining sexual desire, is a gradual process with disappointments and setbacks. The key is to remain on the same intimate team and see revitalized sexuality as a victory over sexual trauma. The give-and-take of intimate sexuality ultimately overcame the rape incident.

LEARNING YOUR CHILD HAD BEEN SEXUALLY ABUSED

Parents fear something negative happening to the child, and if it does, blame themselves. The fear is compounded if the incident involves sexual abuse, especially if the perpetrator is an adult the parents knew and trusted.

When you learn your child has been sexually abused, the focus from the beginning is helping the child to be a survivor rather than a stigmatized victim. First, help her accept the complex reality of the abuse, with all the attendant thoughts and feelings (negative and positive, rational and irrational). Second, listen to her in a caring manner—what she is feeling, what happened, and what help she wants from you. Third, be clear that the responsibility for the abuse lies with the perpetrator, not the child. She need not blame herself or feel guilty. Fourth, the child deserves the understanding, support, and help of family, friends, school, community, counselors, and police. Fifth, this traumatic event is a challenge to provide positive sexuality education. Last, and most important, the child acknowledges that she coped and survived. Her self-esteem is that of a survivor and winner, not a victim and loser. A favorite adage is, "Living well is the best revenge." She emerges from the abusive incident as a resilient, aware child who will make sexuality a positive part of her growing up and adulthood.

Fran and Joshua

A popular folk saying is, "When it rains, it pours." Within a six-month period; Joshua was laid off and since then working as a temp, Fran's mother was diagnosed with liver cancer, Fran and Joshua's twelve-year-old daughter had a broken leg, and Joshua's brother separated from his wife. The biggest stress was learning that the church youth leader had sexually abused eight boys, one of them their son. They had discussed sexual abuse with the two older daughters, but not with their nine-year-old-son. They believed the cultural myth that boys were not victims of childhood sexual abuse.

Jordan did not want to talk about the sexual incident. He felt ashamed, he thought he had done something wrong and caused the abuse. Boys have to deal with a triple stigma: (1) abuse is supposed to happen to girls, not boys; (2) because it's a same-sex incident, the stigma and fear of homosexuality; (3) males are supposed to be strong and streetwise, so he must be weak and deficient. In addition Jordan had to deal with the very public dispute in the church community. The youth leader had been well liked by both the boys and adults on the church board. Jordan did not want the youth leader to lose his job or go to jail. Jordan felt the adults were angry at him. Our culture tends to "blame the victim," and this tendency is at its worst in sexual abuse of boys. There was tremendous confusion about the sexual incidents. The abusive behavior consisted of manually and orally stimulating the boys, usually in a group situation. Jordan found it exciting, got an erection, but didn't ejaculate, although some of the boys did. What did this mean? Was he homosexual? Was he not masculine enough? Why didn't he ejaculate?

Disclosure of the sexual abuse left Jordan confused, anxious, depressed, and filled with guilt and shame. He blamed himself in small and large ways. He wanted to minimize the abuse and remain silent for fear of making things worse. Joshua and Fran didn't know what to do, so they consulted a family therapist with a subspecialty in sexual abuse. She discovered that Jordan liked to draw and tell stories, so they worked together on creating a child's book on sexual abuse. It began with a chapter on normal sexuality for ages eight to twelve, the next chapter was on the myths and "dumb things" people believed about sexuality. Then came a chapter about the sexual incidents with the youth leader—what was special about the experiences and what was confusing, negative, and harmful. The next chapter was what Jordan wanted to happen. Like most children involved in sexual abuse, Jordan wanted to understand the abusive incidents, not feel blamed, and for the abuse to stop. Jordan didn't want anything bad to happen to the youth leader, but wanted him to never abuse any other boys. In the last chapter, Jordan talked about how he was going to be a survivor. When he grew up he planned to help people so they didn't hurt children.

Fran and Joshua joined the therapy sessions and learned how to be good sex educators for Jordan (and his sisters). Sex education shouldn't focus on negatives, STDs/AIDS and sexual abuse. Instead first present a solid base of positive information about sexual development, healthy touch, self-exploration and masturbation, male-female relationships, the importance of love and marriage. His sisters attended one of the family therapy sessions, which ended with a family hug. Joshua and Fran were "askable parents" as well as loving and affectionate with each other and their children. Although everyone wished the sexual abuse had never happened, Fran and Joshua and their children had learned from this experience. Jordan had healed, and they were proud to be a resilient, healthy family. Fran and Joshua worked as a parental team in Jordan's healing process.

CLOSING THOUGHTS

The best way to deal with sexual trauma is prevention. However, bad things do happen to good people. If trauma occurs, don't deny or minimize nor elevate the traumatic incident to control your life and sexual self-esteem. You need to deal with it so you accept the reality, acknowledge you coped and survived, learn from this, and see yourself as a proud survivor. Don't define yourself by the trauma—it's something that happened to you, but does not define you. Psychologically and sexually, "living well is the best revenge." Healing and being resilient is a couple task.

16
EFFECTS OF ROLES AND RESPONSIBILITIES
ON SEXUALITY

A neighbor remarked after reading initial drafts of this manuscript that it sounded great, but didn't describe marriages she was familiar with. "Typical psychologist," she said, "talking about the way things should be, not the way they are."

Consumers have legitimate complaints about self-help books. The guidelines are too glib, the people in the case studies too self-sufficient, things turn out perfectly, people have their cake and eat it too. Self-help books err in being Pollyannaish, promising that if you follow their easy 1-2-3 rules you can have a perfect life, marriage and sex. But couples err on the negative side, settling for too little intimacy and sexual satisfaction in their marriage.

It is possible to fulfill your roles and responsibilities while enjoying a sexually satisfying marriage. You don't need to choose between being a responsible parent, employee, neighbor and church member and being an intimate spouse. These life components can and should complement each other. Research proves that happily married people enjoy and do better in their careers than those with poor marital and/or family relationships.

Married couples, especially those in their middle years, feel burdened by responsibilities. Society depends on middle-years people to be productive as well as care for younger and older generations. Financially, the middle years are the most lucrative, and middle-years people have the most power and influence in our culture. The trade-off is they have the most responsibilities— to their children, the community, jobs, home, and elderly parents. With multiple roles, life is more complex and demanding than when you were a child or young adult.

People who view their roles and responsibilities as burdens, either to be shucked off in becoming liberated or as unending pressures that must be carried through for the good of the family and society but to the detriment of the person, fall into the trap of resentment and blaming. The result is decreased personal, marital and sexual satisfaction. It is healthier to view responsibilities as creative challenges that at times are burdensome and energy-draining but, on the whole, enhance the meaning and quality of your life. This attitude facilitates marital and sexual satisfaction. You needn't make yes-or-no choices between the joys of pleasure-oriented sexuality and responsibilities which include attention to parenting, being a conscientious worker, religious practice, and being a home-oriented person. Your life and marriage are healthier if you view sexuality as integral to the marital bond. Congruence among attitudes, behavior, and feelings enhances psychological well-being and marital satisfaction.

Contrary to popular mythology, couples who have positive, non-repressive, non-guilt driven religious beliefs enjoy better marriages and marital sex. It is erroneously believed that the more religious a person is, the less sexually satisfied he is. Recent data indicates just the opposite. Religious people report greater marital and sexual satisfaction than nonreligious couples.

Erica and Don

Erica and Don were involved with a church-sponsored couples' reading and discussion group. A prime focus was changes in their lives and responsibilities during sixteen years of marriage.

Erica had dropped out of college, left home, and was working in a furniture store when she met Don. Don was from a conservative background and returned to his parents' home after completing college. His goal was to save money and open his own business. At thirty-eight he was the owner of a successful sporting goods store. Erica had stayed home with the children, now thirteen and ten, until they'd begun school. Then she returned to college, finished her degree, obtained a master's, and recently was promoted to physical therapy supervisor. With two children, two careers, two cars, and a house, Don and Erica had a busy and full life.

Nevertheless, they worried about the direction of their life. Did the way they lived reflect their values or were they simply stumbling along day to day? At the birth of their first child, they resumed church attendance. Their church group read about and discussed issues of values and the meaning of life. Sexually, they were a functional couple, but in the past few years there had been a subtle decrease in spontaneity and pleasure in lovemaking. Like so many couples in their middle years, when they talked about sex, they did not talk about their sexuality but concerns about adolescent sexuality and political arguments about sexual values and behavior in America.

Their church group read books on spirituality and the meaning of life. On their own Erica and Don read about the role of sex and marriage. Some of the ideas, such as watching pornographic videos, struck them as immoral. Others, like sanctioned extra-marital affairs and open sharing of details, seemed self-defeating and unrealistic. Still others—weekends away at resorts—were just not appealing. Concepts that focused on enhancing intimacy such as permission to enjoy couple time without feeling guilty, use of multiple stimulation during intercourse, spending ten minutes on afterplay, were appealing and incorporated into their lives. It is okay to leave business calls unreturned for an hour, not volunteer for another community ad hoc committee, not be the parent who drives the kids to every Saturday soccer game. To Erica and Don, spirituality meant a sense of family and religious connection and a feeling of inner peace and meaning. They set aside time after church to play doubles tennis, go to Sunday brunch, and discuss couple and family issues.

Like other middle-years couples, Don and Erica had ''a lot of balls in the air.'' As is true for many couples, it was the ''sexual ball'' that was easiest to drop. Erica emphasized enhancing intimacy, especially incorporating nondemand pleasuring. For that to happen she had to take a break from the frenzied pace of the day. She needed time by herself to relax before being with Don. High on Erica's list of priorities was attending to the needs of their children—she was distressed by the number of ''latchkey children'' in the neighborhood. This meant paying attention to the children's physical needs and getting them from place to place, but more importantly listening to them, being genuinely interested in their activities and projects, and knowing their friends. How could conflicting needs for attention to children and for individual and couple time be met?

On nights when Don and Erica planned to be sexual, Erica would spend time with the children before and during dinner. After dinner she would read, sew, or take a relaxing bath. Don took charge of homework, activities, and getting the kids ready for bed. Instead of waiting until late to start, Don met Erica in the bedroom at nine-thirty. They began by talking and caressing instead of immediately starting sexual stimulation. This was pleasuring time, not goal-oriented foreplay. Their talks and looks served as psychological seduction which, combined with non-demand pleasuring, built sexual anticipation.

At church and in their discussion group, people talked of marriage as a sacrament. A good marriage and loving family was conceptualized as a religious vocation. Intellectually, that sounded good, but what about sex within marriage? Sexuality issues were particularly difficult for Don. He enjoyed receiving oral sex because it was special and exciting. When Erica talked about how much she enjoyed receiving oral sex, Don had uneasy, hard to articulate feelings. Receiving so much pleasure from an act that was not described in the Bible and did not involve the union of man and woman felt sinful. Intellectually Don accepted the view of "God as love" (as opposed to God righteously punishing sinners) and objected to religion's traditional role of inhibiting the expression of pleasure. However, it was not easy for him to integrate sexual expression with religious beliefs. Feelings do not change just because attitudes change or you try something new; change and integration is an ongoing process. Emotional openness, sharing erotic feelings, and valuing intimate sexuality facilitated integration of sexuality and spirituality in Don and Erica's marriage.

ROLES AND RESPONSIBILITIES

In the stereotype of the traditional family, the roles of men and women are clearly delineated and entirely separate. The male's roles are instrumental: bring home money, discipline children, do home repairs, be head of the family. The woman's roles are nurturing: care for children, cook and clean so your husband can relax, service him sexually, maintain a loving family, and be sure everyone's (except your own) emotional needs are taken care of.

We try to confront these cultural stereotypes in our marriage. We strive to make our marital roles equitable. Each of us has skills and interests, we don't split tasks fifty-fifty. The "liberated" concept of everything being shared equally is rigid and unrealistic.

We emphasize equity in power and task distribution rather than fifty-fifty equality. Each person has his/her competencies and interests, and there is role flexibility. Flexible does not mean chaotic. For a family to operate, there has to be structure and role assignments; each person takes responsibility for significant tasks. Sharing roles and responsibilities involves willingness to negotiate and reach agreements. Identify your interests and competencies and use this as a basis for choosing tasks instead of obeying stereotypically masculine or feminine role prescriptions. Remain flexible, even the best thought-out system has glitches. Humor is the best antidote to power struggles and frustrations.

Sometimes tasks involve a reversal of traditional roles. For example, Emily is mechanically skilled and takes prime responsibility for household repairs, whereas Barry enjoys doing dishes and is responsible for kitchen cleanup. Discipline of the children was shared, as was caring for and nurturing them. Providing a parental model of flexibly sharing tasks is an excellent way for children to learn about male-female roles.

Money is a major issue in almost all marriages. No matter how much you have, it never seems enough for all your responsibilities and desires. In the worst of situations, the man complains that his only function is to "bring home the bacon," and berates the wife for spending money. The woman may feel emotionally abandoned by the spouse, who values his job over their marriage and family. She takes satisfaction from accumulating material goods—at the same time indirectly getting back at the husband, who does not satisfy her needs for companionship and intimacy. This is a trap too many couples fall into. Money issues are among the most stressful and disruptive in marriage.

Guidelines for sexual communication are relevant when communicating about financial matters. Each couple has to develop its own money-management style, depending on background, circumstances, habits, and values. You will manage better if you view money as a couple issue with joint responsibility for decisions. When you are honest with each other about how much money is earned, where and for what it is spent, and make requests of how to allocate money, financial issues can be dealt with in a productive manner.

One definite "no-no" is a trade-off between money and sex (we're not talking about prostitution). Don't fall into the trap of saying, "If we have sex this special way, I'll buy you a winter coat," or being angry about a money issue and refusing to have sex until you get your way. Marriages in which sex is used as a financial bargaining chip run a high risk of major problems. When you play a power game with money, no one wins. The marital bond is the ultimate loser.

The three issues that engender the most tension are money, sex and children. Couples talk about sex with a therapist much more readily than they reveal their financial affairs. Handling money responsibly is a difficult task. Couples who develop a successful money management system have a major marital resource.

PARENTING

Parenting children is a major role and responsibility. That is why we emphasize the importance of planned, wanted children. In many ways the ages of your children are more important than your age in terms of how you organize your life.

Roles and responsibilities change dramatically according to the age of the child. The stresses and joys of parenting a baby are quite different from those you experience with a toddler, which in turn are quite different with a preschooler. When you send the child to school you feel relief from the constant responsibilities, but are faced with new ones—interacting with teachers, school officials, community athletic teams, music or dance instructors, coordinating play activities with other parents. Couples hope that as children become older they will require less time and energy, but that's not true. Parenting changes in terms of skills and roles, but at every stage being a parent is a time-consuming and challenging task. During the golden years of childhood, ages seven to eleven, children want and need guidance, support, and time from parents.

Parenting an adolescent can be as draining as parenting a baby, except you have more control over babies. A favorite metaphor is the "emotional bank account" theory of parenting. You establish positive bonds with a baby and youngster and gradually accumulate a wealth of small deposits in the parent-child emotional bank account. In adolescence, there are fewer deposits and often many withdrawals, some of them massive. You want to be sure there is a positive balance left at age eighteen.

We believe, theoretically and personally, that parenting is one of life's major challenges and sources of satisfaction. Parenting goes better when the mother and father share roles and responsibilities in an equitable manner. Men learn to change diapers and give emotional support. Women can be disciplinarians and coach sports teams. Develop a style of parenting that fits your interests, skills, and life circumstances. Remember, each child is unique. Because a parenting approach was helpful with one child doesn't mean it will fit the needs of the sibling.

Parents are individual people as well as a married couple with needs for time and privacy. Balancing individual, couple, and parental roles is a complex challenge, but worthwhile for all involved. The husband-wife bond is the most important relationship in the family. If that is functional and satisfying, other family relationships will thrive. In the long run, putting aside time to be an intimate couple facilitates being better parents.

COMMUNICATION ACROSS GENERATIONS

One of the most difficult positions is being in the middle, between your parents and children. This is especially true when the issue is sexual values and behavior. You don't want to be the sexual morality arbitrator. Grandparents castigate parents for being too liberal, that sexually kids and society are "going to the dogs." Sexual communication and understanding is rare between middle-years couples and their parents. This problem is even more severe if aging parents have had a poor sexual relationship or a spouse has died.

The solution is refusing to be the middleman. Encourage

grandchildren and grandparents to talk directly with each other. They probably will not agree, but this communication allows the children to gain a different perspective on the world. They'll get to know their grandparents as people who possess a wealth of experience. Grandparents provide an historical and cultural context, including issues of sex and marriage. Children learn that grandparents adapt and change. Exposure to children and adolescents is of great value to grandparents. The child's desire for knowledge and new perspectives provides a challenging and broadening experience for grandparents. The role of the grandparent is downplayed in contemporary America, but it can be of great value to you and your children.

Your role with both older and younger generations is to provide caring, support, and guidance, yet not feel entirely responsible (this is especially important in regard to aging parents and young adult children). The line between being involved and caring on the one hand, but not overly responsible on the other, is difficult to maintain. Some people begin by being authoritarian and domineering, and then overreact and become permissive and ineffectual. Either way, you don't meet the needs of grandparents or children. A healthier approach is to care, support, and help deal with problems and transitions without falling into the trap of trying to impose your will or feeling totally responsible.

Nowhere is the caring approach more crucial, yet more difficult, than in the area of sexuality. In the "good old days," there was a widely believed myth that there was *one* right way to achieve happiness, and it was the parents' responsibility to teach this to children. Parents were judged to be successes or failures by whether the adult child was successful and married. It was a shock to a parent when two, five, ten, or twenty years later the adult child divorced. Was it the parents' fault? Should the parent feel responsible and assume a burden of guilt for the "failure"? There are three myths imbedded in this:

1. There is only one right way to be happy.
2. Parents are primarily, or even entirely, responsible for the successes or failures of their adult children's marital and sexual lives.
3. A divorce is always a sign of failure.

A rational attitude is that your responsibility as a parent is to love, educate, guide, listen to, and support your children.

It is inappropriate and self-defeating to evaluate yourself as a person or parent by how well children are doing at a given point in their lives. As they become young adults, they assume responsibility for decisions about their lives, including decisions about relationships and sexuality. It is not helpful to them or you to feel guilty about parenting. You will be in a better position to help with the present problem if you don't feel burdened by guilt and regrets from the past.

Nick and Sally

Nick and Sally had a difficult time organizing their lives and priorities. This was a second marriage for both. Sally married at seventeen, had two children, divorced at twenty-three, raised the children alone for nine years, and married Nick at thirty-two. Nick's first marriage was initiated at nineteen when the woman became pregnant. After fourteen years of a bad marriage, alcohol abuse, major career disruptions, and two more children, Nick and his wife had the sense to realize this was not a viable marriage. Four years later, Nick married Sally. Sally's daughters lived with them; Nick's children visited weekends and summers, and during difficult periods would stay longer.

As individuals, Nick and Sally had to get their lives together. This included finding better-paying and more satisfying jobs. Even more important, they had to develop a stable and intimate marital bond. Added to this were the stresses of parenting children and stepchildren. "Blended" families are different from nuclear families. They are more exciting and challenging, but also more complex and stressful.

"The most important relationship is our marital bond" was written out and displayed over Nick and Sally's nightstand. Remembering this got them through rough times. They knew that if they could make their marriage good and keep it good, other issues had a better chance of working out. This strategy had a positive effect on the entire family.

Relationships and strains in blended families are real and complex, requiring awareness of emotional boundaries among family members. This requires tolerance and acceptance of different patterns of thinking and behaving. Babies and young children require much time and attention. Nick and Sally were glad to not have to deal with those responsibilities. There is stress in parenting adolescent children because you are dealing with the transition to being an independent, autonomous person. One adolescent had an unwanted pregnancy she chose to terminate, and an adult child was divorced after two stormy years of marriage.

Nick and Sally decided that in dealing with young adult children the best thing to do was give guidance and support when asked, and provide a model which demonstrated that adults can grow and change. They had a strong commitment to nurturing their marital bond. They were upset by family problems, but tried not to feel guilty or overly responsible for their adult children's lives. They were consistent in their caring and support, willing to listen and give advice when asked, but unwilling to take over for the adult children. This strategy was successful both for their marriage and relationships with their adult children.

A widespread delusion for many couples, including ourselves, is that if only we didn't have so many responsibilities and so many roles to play, life would be perfect. If only we lived on a Caribbean island! Like most "if only" thinking, this gets you nowhere—not to mention that there are a multitude of marital, sexual, and family problems on Caribbean islands.

Make an honest and frank appraisal of how you handle roles and responsibilities. Have you allowed jobs, community projects, or unproductive time—watching soap operas, gossiping on the phone—to dominate your life and interfere with your marriage? If so, you need to reorder personal, couple and family priorities. Usually what is needed is not a total life change, instead, set aside time for yourselves as individuals and as an intimate couple. Some couples need to confront a major issue (for example, drinking, being controlled by your job, depression, alienation, anger at a parent or child, overspending credit cards, filling your life with activities so you avoid the spouse). In these circumstances, you need to commit to a change process. We suggest consulting a therapist rather than trying to do this on your own.

CLOSING THOUGHTS

This chapter is not meant to be Pollyannaish: we are not saying you can meet all personal, couple, sexual, family, career, religious, and community needs with never a compromise. You have to honestly assess how you organize your life and roles and responsibilities. You can set priorities, make hard decisions, and stick to your agreements. Even the best of couples have to negotiate difficult issues and accept imperfect agreements. What should not be compromised is couple time and intimacy. Treating yourself well and taking time to be an intimate couple allows you to handle roles and responsibilities instead of seeing them as a burden you resent. Vital sexuality is good for you as a person and your marital bond. It energizes you to deal with roles and responsibilities and facilitates a better quality of life. Feeling good about your marriage and sexuality will pay long-term dividends for parenting, job, and extended family relationships.

17

A COST-BENEFIT ANALYSIS OF EXTRAMARITAL AFFAIRS

Couples read the title of this chapter and are tempted to skip it. They would rather not think about or discuss, much less deal with, the issue of extramarital affairs. The reality is that an extramarital affair by one or both spouses occurs in almost forty percent of American marriages. It is an almost universal experience for both women and men to fantasize about extramarital sex. Our culture provides ample opportunity to engage in or at least consider extramarital relationships. Even former President Carter admitted to lustful thoughts about women. This chapter is not for just a small minority of errant spouses; the issues raised affect the great majority of couples.

No matter what you read in pop psychology books or hear on talk shows, extramarital sex is not an open-and-shut issue. The meaning and impact of an extramarital affair must be understood in the context of the individuals and their marital relationship. An affair could be a strategy for leaving a fatally flawed marriage or an impulsive one-time fling; it might serve as a way of preserving a marriage in which sex is nonexistent or a means of venting anger; it may be an expression of an individual need or a way of gaining the approval of the "boys" during an out-of-town convention; a way to get back at a spouse or a means of trying to make up for feelings of failure; a way to bring romance and excitement into an otherwise depressed life. Each affair has its reasons, its unique set of characteristics, and consequences for the individual and marital bond. Extramarital affairs are an excellent example of how multicausal and multidimensional human sexuality is.

We will not engage in abstract arguments about the rights or wrongs of extramarital sex. Instead, we'll discuss marriages in which affairs occurred and explore how couples dealt with them. We also present guidelines for preventing affairs for couples who make the commitment to marital fidelity.

A common myth about extramarital affairs is that they occur after ten or twenty years of marriage and reflect boredom and a need for variety. In truth, the most common time for an extramarital affair is the first three years of marriage.

TYPES OF AFFAIRS

Extramarital relationships are very complex; be aware of this complexity when thinking about your affair or the spouse's. Arbitrarily, we divide affairs into three categories:

1. High opportunity-low involvement affair—characterized by impulsiveness, little emotional connection, and often paid (massage parlor, prostitute). This is the most common type of male affair.
2. Ongoing affair—a continuous relationship largely sexual as opposed to emotionally based, enjoyable but not committed, not a direct threat to the marriage.
3. Comparison affair—this relationship meets significant sexual and/or emotional needs not met by the marriage. It could be a one-year, ongoing love affair or a highly charged three-week relationship. People end their marriages because of comparison affairs. This is the most common type of female affair.

The male-female double standard greatly influences how people feel about and react to affairs. The traditional double standard holds that males can play around as long as they don't get the woman pregnant, contract a sexually transmitted disease, or fall in love, but the woman must remain faithful. Extramarital affairs somewhat follow this pattern—approximately 20–30 percent of men have an affair sometime during their marriages, most of which are high opportunity and considered of minimal importance. Approximately 15–20 percent of women have affairs, which last longer and are emotionally involving. On two grounds, wives' affairs have more impact on the marriage:

1. They diverge from the double standard and are more distressing for the spouse.
2. A comparison affair is a serious threat to the marriage.

TRAPS IN DISCLOSING AFFAIRS

The pop psychology concepts of "open marriage" and "honestly communicating all details and feelings" are inappropriate and destructive. Although the concept of open marriage was greeted with intellectual excitement and, for a time, became chic, empirical evidence strongly indicates that it is not a functional model for extramarital affairs. An extramarital affair entered into to fulfill the individual's needs might best be dealt with by not sharing specifics with the spouse. Revealing feelings and details is not being open and honest, but a means of expressing hostility or ridding yourself of guilt. It serves to get feelings off your chest while burdening the spouse with doubt, questions about sexual inadequacy, and a need to react. Ask yourself why you are "telling all" and whether your spouse really wants to know all. If you thought out your motivations and sense the spouse does want to know, then by all means share all. Be sure you discuss the affair with a constructive purpose, not a vindictive "let me tell you who it was, exactly how we did it, and how many orgasms we had" manner.

One danger in not informing the spouse is she may find out in an embarrassing or traumatic manner. If the affair was motivated by a problem in the marriage, the spouse is still in the dark about your dissatisfaction. It makes more sense to confront the dissatisfaction directly rather than express it indirectly through an affair.

Whether the affair is ongoing or has been terminated is crucial. It is easier to talk about and deal with an affair that has ended. At some level of awareness, spouses *do* know about the affair, although at first they may react with shock, hurt, and insist they never suspected. On closer examination, it becomes evident that there were clues and dissatisfactions the spouse ignored or discounted. Even the children are aware something has been going on in their parents' marriage.

HOW TO DEAL WITH A REVEALED AFFAIR

People have different feelings, values, and experiences regarding extramarital affairs. If the marriage is to be viable, the revealed affair must be dealt with. Dealing with it can mean anything from having one emotional discussion to entering marriage therapy and discussing feelings of hurt, anger, vulnerability and trust for a year or longer. Typically, dealing with the affair involves a series of emotional interactions—tears, anger, threats—followed by rational discussions of the affair and its meaning. The couple discusses the causes of and feelings about the affair and comes to an explicit agreement regarding future extramarital relationships.

A helpful guideline is to focus on the marriage rather than the affair. Dealing with an affair means discussing marital dissatisfaction with concrete plans to revitalize your intimate bond. It does not mean continually going over details of the affair. One way of viewing an affair is as a cry for help from a marriage that is struggling. If the message is attended to and the crisis dealt with, the marital bond becomes resilient and stronger. Certainly there are more direct and less stressful ways to convey the message. However, if an affair has occurred, it does little good to blame, induce guilt, wallow in self-righteousness, or engage in "if only" thinking. If you choose to revitalize the marriage, focus communication on rebuilding marital and sexual vitality.

This guideline is particularly relevant if the affair remains unknown to the spouse. If you choose to revitalize the marriage, the crucial first step is to end the affair. This is more complex and considerably harder than it sounds. Affairs are easier to get into than out of. You have to free yourself from the affair in order to have the focus and emotional energy to revitalize your intimate bond.

It is true that an extramarital affair heightens the probability the marriage will end in divorce. It is not true that extramarital affairs are the chief cause of divorce. Typically, the problems that precipitated the affair—neglect of the spouse and relationship, sex, money, individual dissatisfaction, childrearing issues—are what cause the marriage to disintegrate, rather than the affair. Affairs are harmful for marriages, but are not the major cause of marital dissolution.

Some people use an affair as a way of getting out of a poor

marriage and/or a transition to being single again. Some marriages cannot recover from an affair. If respect and trust cannot be restored, trying to "save" the marriage is a hopeless task.

Doreen and Al

Doreen and Al were in their late forties. Four years ago their marriage, already in a stressful phase, had been badly shaken by the revelation of Doreen's affair. Al's business was in decline and the money from Doreen's job, which had gone toward house furnishings and vacations, was needed for ongoing expenses. Doreen was resentful that Al didn't ask for or acknowledge her financial aid during this crisis.

Al denied he was depressed, avoided talking about problems, drank heavily, stayed out late, and had a brief sexual fling (high opportunity-low involvement affair). Doreen was being sexually ignored, and suspected Al was having a number of affairs. He was paying little attention to the children, which put a further burden on Doreen. Previously, when Al was depressed, drinking, and staying away from the family, she passively accepted his behavior. This time her resentment peaked, and she rebelled against being at his beck and call.

Doreen was happy to receive attention from a buyer at work, and within three weeks embarked on a passionate affair (a comparison affair). Doreen loved the attention of a younger man who found her sexually attractive. They went to gourmet restaurants and had sex at fashionable hotels. Al was so self-involved, he didn't notice how often Doreen was gone or that the kids' needs were being ignored. This situation continued for five months. It was twelve-year-old Gordy's arrest for shoplifting that brought the issue to a head. Al ranted and raved, demanding to know why Doreen didn't supervise the children and where she had been. Doreen said she wasn't putting up with him any more and was leaving, at which time a very ugly scene ensued, with name-calling, pushing, and threats.

Doreen found the lover relationship easier when it was an affair, not a substitute for marriage. The affair began to sour after she left Al. The young man did not want to deal with Doreen's feelings of confusion, anger and guilt or her children. Al was feeling even worse. His business, marriage, and relationship with his children were all going to hell, he felt lonely and unable to cope. Although many people would have sought therapy at this time (before the crisis would have been more appropriate), Al and Doreen were stubborn enough to keep the situation in this intolerable holding pattern for another two months.

It was Al who made the first move toward reconciliation. He sold the business and began working for a colleague. Al felt a strong need to get his life together; for him that meant reestablishing the security of marriage and family. He resented Doreen's affair, but very much wanted her back. Doreen did not enjoy being separated, but was reluctant to reenter a marriage in which there were financial problems, resentment, and Al's history of depression, noncommunication, and alcohol abuse. Yet she couldn't turn her back on eighteen years of marriage and reject Al's request to make a good faith effort to revitalize their marital bond.

Before resuming living together, Doreen and Al had serious conversations about their marriage and the issue of affairs. Doreen refused to be the "bad guy," although she did regret, and apologized for, her affair. They recommitted to marital fidelity. This is the most common agreement for couples who are trying to rebuild their marital bond. Al agreed to talk things over when he was upset instead of ignoring Doreen and drinking to excess. Al's business problems caused marital conflict. When there would be business and financial stress, Al agreed to use positive coping techniques like exercise, meditation, taking walks with Doreen, and talking about concerns. He committed to abstaining from alcohol when there was work-related stress, agreeing to drink only in social situations.

Four years later, their life was on solid footing, partly because they were doing better financially and working at jobs they liked. They valued their marriage and sexual relationship and devoted time and attention to it. Successfully dealing with the crisis made them feel better about themselves as people and strengthened the intimate bond. They felt better prepared to be parents of adolescents, which can put stress on the most stable marriage.

OUTCOMES OF AFFAIRS

Anger, guilt, confusion, and distrust are emotions people typically attach to extramarital affairs. Envy, a sense of excitement, heightened sexual desire, and an appreciation of spontaneity are also possible outcomes. Couples whose sex lives have been mediocre or nonexistent for years report a sexual reawakening. Instead of taking the spouse for granted and being satisfied with the same old marital sex, there is renewed sexual interest and desire. Couple sex becomes creative and satisfying.

Joe and Gail

Joe and Gail were thought of as the perfect couple. They liked and respected each other, enjoyed doubles tennis and hosting dinner parties, were involved parents who loved their children, supported each other in their careers, and had an easy, affectionate relationship. Yet their sex life had always been disappointing. At best, intercourse frequency was once a week. Joe would initiate in a clumsy, goal-oriented manner and ejaculated quickly. Occasionally, Gail would be orgasmic, but this was rare, more a pleasant surprise than an integral part of sexual responsivity.

Joe enrolled in a six-week managerial training program and, during the first week, was seduced by one of the trainers. It was an amazing sexual five weeks. Joe was introduced to oral sex, which increased his receptivity to penile stimulation and facilitated development of ejaculatory control. She taught Joe how to stimulate a woman and he learned it was normal and expected for the partner to be orgasmic. When Joe returned home, he had to decide how to convey his newfound sexual interest and competence.

Joe chose not to reveal details, but told Gail he wanted to improve the quality of their sexual relationship. Gail surmised he'd had an affair, but chose not to pursue the issue. She was receptive and pleased by his new sexual comfort and skill. The best kind of an affair is one that is totally separate from the marriage. Within five months, they developed a satisfying couple sexual style. Joe was no longer looking back on the affair, but enjoying a creative, playful sexual relationship with his wife. Gail was more responsive and orgasmic than ever before. With the help of learning from the affair, marital sex was an energizing component of their bond, not a source of frustration and discontent. They were building a reservoir of shared intimacy. The implicit agreement was not to discuss Joe's affair, an appropriate choice for them. Gail made it clear her openness was based on Joe's commitment to fidelity. Gail and Joe valued marital sex and the security of their intimate bond.

John and Helen

John and Helen's experience with integrating an affair is particularly enlightening. They'd been married twenty-three years. Early in the marriage, while John was in the service, both had brief affairs; these were never discussed. Shortly after the marriage of their oldest son, John began an affair with a young, single woman at work. This affair continued on an intermittent basis over three years, causing a good deal of disruption in the marriage and for the adolescent daughter living at home.

John felt this was his last chance to make a significant change in his life. The affair offered sexual variety and excitement. John was motivated by a need to reaffirm vitality and reassert control over his life. Throughout this period, he continued to care for Helen, although there was a good deal of hurt and anger. Helen was not a martyr, but chose not to force John to leave the house. She dealt with her feelings by discussing issues with friends and putting energy into her job. She continued active involvement in parenting as well as activities and projects that affirmed her self-worth.

After John's affair ran its course, Helen and John spent three weeks at a quiet beach. There was no dramatic Hollywood reconciliation, but they did commit to revitalizing their marital bond. Feelings of hurt, vulnerability, resentment, and disappointment did not just vanish. Rather than the popular adage "Forgive and forget," Helen forgave John, but not the behavior—it was "Forgive and remember." John knew Helen would not tolerate another affair.

The healing and rebuilding process occurred over a year's period, and even now there are scars and sensitive areas. Helen resented having to assume the role of prime parent during those three years. John had taken Helen for granted and treated their marital bond in a disrespectful manner.

This marriage had enough strength to weather the storm and turmoil of an affair. John doubts he would have had the emotional strength to maintain the marriage if it was Helen who'd had the affair. In the same way that there are seasons in a person's life, there are seasons in a marriage. John and Helen had a three-year winter, but with a renewed sense of commitment to their intimate bond and willingness to deal with feelings, the relationship again bloomed.

PREVENTION OF AFFAIRS

Most prevention advice is simplistic and moralistic. Extramarital sex is viewed as an evil to be prevented at all costs. This advice ignores the realities, opportunities, and complexities of sexuality in contemporary America. Each marriage is different. Interest in and opportunity for an extramarital affair has to be understood in the context of the marriage, the circumstances, and the individuals involved.

In an ideal scenario, early in the marriage, and even before marriage, the couple would have a frank discussion about the role of marital sexuality and share thoughts and feelings about extramarital affairs. This is seldom, if ever, done. One consequence is the couple sitting in a therapist's office dealing with the crisis of a discovered affair. Each person had a different implicit assumption about affairs. Typically, the woman's assumption is that there will not be an affair. She feels particularly vulnerable if it was she who had the affair. The man's assumption is that he can have brief or discreet affairs—no harm done if it "doesn't mean anything." He's shaken by the marital crisis caused by his affair. No one plans to have a comparison affair.

A good guideline is: the better the marriage, the more reason to decide against an extramarital affair. It is too disruptive and draining, not worth putting a satisfying relationship under stress. Prevention is the most cost-efficient strategy.

Perhaps the best prevention technique is to have a clear understanding about the type of affair each partner is vulnerable to, and how to avoid falling into an affair. For example, women who are friendly and touchers are vulnerable for a male friendship turning into a sexual affair. A coping strategy would be for the husband to meet the men she works with or serves on committees with. She clearly states she is gregarious, but has a strong sense of marital loyalty. Potential affairs thrive on secrecy and intrigue. This strategy makes feelings and expectations clear.

Males are particularly vulnerable to high opportunity-low involvement affairs. There is a great deal of peer pressure to have one-night stands, go to a massage parlor or a prostitute. Saying no is not part of the male role, he's considered a wimp. He needs to talk this through with his wife so there is an active coping strategy which allows him to avoid these situations or assertively say he's not interested. For people who travel a great deal or are in ''high opportunity for affairs jobs''—salesmen, musicians, police officers, athletes, or teachers—it is important to have a safe agenda such as working out, reading or writing, calling home, having a project or hobby while on the road. Boredom as well as secrecy provides a fertile breeding ground for affairs. Spouses commit to talk out a high risk situation rather than feeling embarrassed or guilty, keeping this secret for fear of alarming the spouse.

Another strategy is an agreement to tell the spouse you are considering having an affair before acting on it. In movies, novels, and especially soap operas, people are swept away by impulsive, uncontrollable urges. Our guidelines would not make a good plot line for a movie, but does make for a resilient trust bond in a marriage. The spouse cannot force or coerce you to remain faithful. Respect for the spouse is strong enough that you keep the agreement to talk to him before acting on a desire to have an affair. It will be a stressful and confrontative talk, but one that forces each spouse to examine how an affair will impact his/her life. It promotes discussion of the risks of STDs/HIV and pregnancy, as well as the threat to marital intimacy.

A different level of prevention occurs after an extramarital affair, when the choice is to revitalize the marriage. Discuss the meaning of the affair, and more important, how to deal with the aftermath so this does not dominate your marriage. Trust is the element most disrupted by an extramarital affair. If the marriage is to be revitalized, you need to restore trust by making a clear agreement concerning future affairs. Most couples choose abstinence from affairs and put their energy into rebuilding the intimacy bond.

The extramarital affair need not be a "hot," supersensitive topic. Avoid the extremes of denial or obsessive focus. Life, sex, and marriage are meant to be lived in the present, not controlled by memories/grudges from the past or fearful obsessing about the future. When an affair has occurred, learn from it. What was being communicated by the affair and what should you attend to in your lives and marriage? The best prevention strategy is to keep the marital bond of respect, trust, and intimacy strong and vital.

In discussing these examples, we are not encouraging couples to experiment with extramarital affairs. Certainly, we are not saying that what every marriage needs is an affair to reawaken emotional and sexual feelings. In our marriage, we have chosen—and it has been a conscious and discussed choice—not to have affairs. This decision comes from awareness that trust and intimacy would be disrupted, although we do not believe it would be destroyed, by an affair.

OUR MARITAL AGREEMENT

We discussed a number of crucial issues before marrying. We reached agreements about contraception and planning children, where we would live, careers, money, and dealing with extended family. A notable area we did not discuss was sexuality and extramarital affairs. In retrospect, we had the typical anxieties and inhibitions of other young couples. As our relationship progressed, we had open conversations about sexuality, making requests, and improving the quality of marital sex. However, we studiously avoided discussion of extramarital affairs.

The topic came up in a serendipitous fashion. A mutual friend, a male teaching assistant, had a female student who was flunking. She approached him and offered to do anything he wanted Saturday night if she could only pass the course. The teaching assistant was both ethical and "uptight," and told her what she needed to do was stay home and study. This story was greeted with great laughter. Afterward Emily asked Barry what he would do if a young woman approached him. Barry tried his best to avoid dealing with the question, but Emily insisted they talk this out. She wanted to understand his viewpoint and feelings. Barry assured her that if he had an affair it would be totally separate from the marriage and would just be a fun fling for excitement and variety. This was Barry's implicit assumption about extramarital affairs, but it sounded strange when made explicit. Emily was adamant that if Barry had an option to have affairs, then to maintain a sense of equity, she wanted the same option. She was not interested in a high opportunity affair or a quick fling, but would want a sense of involvement. Barry was upset, and said this kind of affair would be a threat to their marriage. Emily replied if they were going to have an agreement about affairs, it had to be an equitable one.

We agreed that neither of us would have an affair. The advantage of talking about issues and making an explicit agreement is that the guidelines are clear. The disadvantage is, if one or both spouses break the agreement you will need to confront feelings of disappointment and anger. He can't say it wasn't a big deal or he didn't know.

Our agreement has worked well for us. We aren't worried when one travels or goes to dinner or a meeting with a friend of the opposite sex. This is how we've chosen to deal with the issue of extramarital affairs, but it does not mean it is the right choice for you. Each couple needs to consider their situation, marriage, and values and choose what is in their best interest. This is our decision rather than the "right" one. We do not want to convey a "holier than thou" attitude.

CLOSING THOUGHTS

Couples engage in extramarital affairs for different reasons. The affair can have both helpful and harmful effects on the marriage. The resolution of the affair and how it is dealt with varies greatly among individuals and couples. There is not "one right way" to handle the issue of extramarital sex. It is normal to experience a range of feelings and reactions. The theme of this chapter is that, contrary to social pronouncements, people do have extramarital affairs and these can be dealt with if the couple is motivated. An extramarital affair strains the trust bond, but need not break it. If the marriage is to be vital and satisfying, you have to put time and energy into rebuilding respect, trust, intimacy, and sexuality.

18
SEX IN SECOND MARRIAGES

Marriage is not easy. Remarriage is a special challenge, a commitment to create a satisfying and stable relationship free of the bitterness and pain of the first. Folk wisdom has it that "There is no gathering the rose without being pricked by the thorns."

When you marry, you do so with the hope that this marriage will be satisfying and enduring: "Love 'til the twelfth of never." For almost fifty percent of couples, this hope becomes a statistic—a divorce statistic. The failure of that marriage doesn't mean you are a failure or a second marriage would be unwise. Choosing to divorce can be a sign of psychological health and good judgment. Feeling you are a failure because of divorce is not rational. You are not a failure as a person, a sexual being, or a partner for a second marriage.

There are many reasons for divorce, the foremost being that the marriage was entered into for the wrong reasons and/or you chose an inappropriate partner. Other causes are: the couple were not ready for a marital commitment, children born too soon put too much stress on the relationship, or as the people matured, one changed in ways to which the marital relationship could not adapt. Divorce might follow as a reaction to an extramarital affair or because the couple simply grew apart. Some marriages are "fatally flawed." Just as each marriage is unique, so are the reasons for dissolving it.

The primary reason for the increased divorce rate is that divorce is now accepted as a viable alternative to a marginal or destructive marriage. Traditionally, there were strong family, religious, and societal pressures to remain married even if the marriage was a disaster for the individuals and children. These external "glues" kept poor, unsatisfying marriages intact, resulting in dysfunctional, disturbed families. In the 1990s, the marital bond needs to be strong and vital. People have better-quality marriages than a generation ago. There is also more marital dissolution. Marriages that survived because of external supports and the stigma of divorce do not survive in the 1990s. But is that really a loss?

Be aware of the causes for the dissolution of the first marriage. This is not to punish yourself or consider the marriage a failure, but to learn from the experience. What you learn about yourself and what you value in a relationship will help you choose a second marriage that will be satisfying and enduring. The great majority of both men and women remarry. Second marriages which are successful (the divorce rate is higher in second marriages) are happier and more sexually fulfilling. This is true if you learned from the first experience, chose better, and put time and psychological energy into the marriage to make it satisfying and secure.

Susan

Susan married at nineteen, bore two children, separated at twenty-six, divorced at twenty-eight, and, after a series of relationships, was considering remarriage at thirty-four. From her first experience she learned that marriage was not the answer for other problems, such as a desire to leave home or uncertainty about vocational goals. Susan knew she was capable of living independently, enjoyed mothering, and realized she did not have to be married in order to function personally, financially or sexually. In assessing the first marriage, Susan knew she did not want to marry a man who drank heavily and spent more time with the boys than with his wife and family. Susan liked active men who were ambitious and did not want to stay in the same house and job all their lives. She wanted a man who was willing to be an involved stepfather and interested in having a second family.

Her years as a single-again woman had been painful and isolated at times, yet worthwhile. Susan's self-esteem improved, although her relationships were not particularly rewarding, either sexually or emotionally. She had not deceived herself into thinking otherwise. Susan was planful, choiceful, and assertive in organizing her life. If she remarried, she wanted a partner whom she respected, trusted, and with whom she could share emotional and sexual intimacy.

Susan wanted financial security and a father for her children. Her first husband rarely saw the children. But these were not the most important factors in the decision to marry Rick. Susan found in Rick a man who was aware of her emotional and sexual feelings and open to feedback and guidance. The critical factor for Susan was Rick's willingness to commit the time and energy to develop a satisfying, secure intimate bond.

Susan's second marriage was successful because of her awareness, sense of personal responsibility, and realization that marriage was a choice, not a mandate. Although three of four women and six of seven divorced men eventually remarry (the percentage is lower for widows and widowers and considerably lower for older women), not remarrying is a viable alternative. You can have a successful life—including a sexually functional life—without marriage. The best reason to remarry is the desire to share your life with this person. People remarry because it is expected, for security, to have a parent for their children, or to avoid loneliness. These can be valid and important factors, but when they are prime motives, it is difficult to choose well. Marrying for negative reasons or unfulfilled needs makes it unlikely you will assess the new partner and relationship realistically. You need to thoughtfully discuss values, goals, feelings, life plans, and your viability as a couple. When motivation is positive, you are more likely to choose well and have a successful second marriage.

The most important guideline is not to play the "comparison game." Start fresh with the new spouse. Nowhere is this truer than in the bedroom. Many people, especially males, believe the myth they know all there is to know about sex because of experiences with the first spouse and/or other partners. Sexually, each person is unique. Be aware of and acknowledge the partner's uniqueness instead of depending on what "worked" with previous partners. Be open to new sexual scenarios and techniques. Establish a feedback system to share what is and isn't comfortable and pleasurable. Developing a couple sexual style takes practice and feedback, but most of all, requires awareness of the necessity to do so.

Ed

Ed had a poor marriage of fifteen years duration. For the first ten years sex was one of the strengths, but this too degenerated when fighting, disillusionment, and bitterness increased. The event that eventually ended the marriage was Ed's discovery of her extramarital affair. Soon after the divorce, she married that man. Ed felt inadequate and obsessively worried he was sexually inferior to the other man.

Two years later, Ed married Ann, who had been divorced for three years. When Ann was assertive and made sexual requests Ed felt threatened, became hostile, and told her if she did not like his way of making love, she could find someone else. Ann began thinking of Ed as an insecure, chauvinistic male. She was doing what self-help books and the women's group she attended recommended. Ann was frustrated that sexual requests weren't working, instead causing a major rift in this marriage, which was particularly galling because her first husband had objected adamantly when she'd learned to stand up for her rights. Ed became angry and defensive when Ann said anything about sexual technique.

Luckily, Ed and Ann were intelligent people, cared about each other, and had enough commitment that they sought marital therapy. The clinician helped them see that negative experiences from their first marriages were interfering with the development of a satisfying sexual bond. Ed's defensiveness was identified and reduced. Ann stated clearly that she loved him and wanted sexuality to be good for *both* of them. With this as a foundation, Ann could make sexual requests and guide Ed. No longer inhibited and insecure, Ed became comfortable and skilled as a lover. With Ann's sensitivity to rejection reduced, she became more sexually responsive. Occasionally as with most couples, they would fall into old traps of being defensive and frustrated. They identified present problems to deal with, and let go of fears and resentments from the past.

Even if a person has thirty years of positive sexual experi-

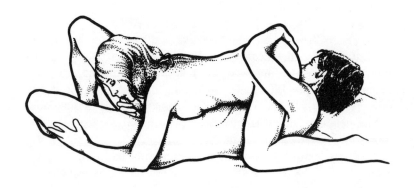

Many couples find mutual oral-genital sex the most arousing kind of multiple stimulation. Each can let go and express their passion.

ences, he needs to come into a second marriage with an open, receptive attitude. Each partner brings both helpful and inhibiting sexual attitudes and skills to a second marriage. To be a sexually functional couple you have to learn together. You develop a unique marital and sexual style. It takes most couples at least six months to create a high-quality, intimate, sexually expressive relationship. This approach is relevant not only to sexual issues but also communication, conflict resolution, satisfactory agreements, and enjoyment of each other.

After being hurt in a first marriage it is extremely difficult for some people to be vulnerable and risk becoming deeply and intimately involved.

Terri

Terri was forty-three years old and still suffering psychological scars from her first marriage. Hers was the classic story of a nurse who marries a young man entering medical school. She gave up her career plans and worked extra jobs so he could finish school and an extended residency program. He was absorbed in completing his training and building a practice. During these years, few of Terri's needs were met. There was little time for the marital relationship to thrive. Most of their sexual contacts were of the ''slam, bam, thank you ma'am'' variety (professional people, including psychologists, fall into this trap too). While the husband grew intellectually and underwent tremendous professional and personal changes, Terri's life stagnated. Her role was to support him financially and give him freedom to pursue his career.

When Terri decided it was time to start a family, he shocked her with the news that he was no longer in love with her. He refused to have a child to shore up their failing marriage, and asked for a divorce. Terri was devastated, felt used, depressed, and attempted suicide. The divorce was bitter, and her subsequent years as a divorcée dealing with the roller coaster of dating relationships further disillusioned and hardened Terri.

In the second marriage, Terri did learn from the mistakes of the first. She had chosen a man who was considerate, caring, and clearly loved her. He did not ask her to give up personal plans, friends, or job. They reached mutually satisfying agreements on how to organize career and couple activities. However, it was extremely difficult for Terri to risk being emotionally vulnerable. She was embittered that at forty-three she felt too old to have a child, angry at having been used and discarded by her first husband, and unwilling to commit to an intimate relationship in which she would once again risk rejection. Because of Terri's reluctance, the husband became less emotionally involved. Her second marriage was vastly superior to the first, yet both Terri and her husband felt cheated because it was not the intimate, emotionally satisfying relationship it could have been.

Trevor

A very different outcome occurred with Trevor, who chose to take risks and make himself vulnerable in his second marriage. He too felt manipulated and devastated by his first marriage. He had married Janie whom he'd known in high school, when she became pregnant the summer after graduation. She had family and psychological problems, and used their marriage and child as a way to feel loved and worthwhile.

Trevor was in the service when he married and in Vietnam when his son was born. By the time he returned home, the marriage was in dire straits. Janie had been unable to tolerate the stress of living alone with a baby and moved in with another man. Trevor persuaded her to return, and they spent three conflict-ridden years attempting to salvage their poorly thought-out marriage. It ended in a bitter divorce. Trevor felt the alimony and child support payments were excessive. Because of ongoing financial conflicts, he did not have regular contact with his son, which depressed him and to his great regret all but destroyed the father-son bond.

Trevor valued the idea of marriage and children. Even though his first experience had been bitter, it did not disillusion him about the intimacy and security possible in marriage. Because of his poor financial situation, he had to move back with his parents and take a second job. It took him over two years to get back on his feet financially and psychologically.

A year and a half later, Trevor began dating Kathy, who was also divorced. Their relationship developed slowly. Trevor and Kathy discussed emotional reactions to their divorces and what it would take for them to be a successful and stable couple. The idealistic, romantic feelings and illusions experienced at twenty are not repeated the second time around, nor should they be. We as a culture are enthralled with the concept of romantic love, but romantic love and passionate sex are not a good basis for partner choice, much less a satisfying and secure marriage. The emotional highs of a dating relationship motivate the person to take risks and increase involvement. Unfortunately, couples are swept away by romantic love and don't discuss personal strengths and weaknesses, nor objectively examine the strengths and potential incompatibilities of their relationship. The advantage people like Trevor and Kathy have is that they're motivated to take a critical look at themselves and the relationship before committing to marriage. You lose romantic mystique, but through a realistic appraisal of yourself, your partner, the relationship and the situation, you gain a marriage with a greater likelihood of success.

Their marriage has been intimate and committed for over ten years. Parenting their eight-year-old daughter has been highly satisfying for Trevor. His divorce and its aftermath were traumatic, but did not so scar him that he wasn't willing to risk again. Trevor and Kathy have one of the best second marriages— or for that matter, *any* marriage—we know of.

GUIDELINES FOR A SECOND MARRIAGE

An open attitude and willingness to commit—the old cliché "nothing ventured, nothing gained"—is crucial to a successful second marriage. Second marriages can be better than intact first marriages. They are most successful when the person has learned from the first experience, carefully and wisely chosen a second spouse, risks being vulnerable, puts energy into the relationship, and is committed to making this marriage successful. The couple shares sexual experiences, is spontaneous and experimental, and aware of and responsive to the spouse's feelings and preferences. It is helpful to state your intentions directly: "I want our marriage to be vital and satisfying. I have a lot to learn about you and you have a lot to learn about me. If we share as a couple, it will be fun. I want to know what makes you feel good, what arouses you, and what you don't like. I have to unlearn things from my first marriage, and I bet you do, too. Let's not be afraid to try. I love you and want sex to nurture and energize our marital bond.''

Sex serves to make special the marital bond and deepen and reinforce intimacy. A couple who is sexually open and vulnerable will generalize these attitudes and feelings to other areas of the marriage. Feeling good about your sexual bond helps to ease the inevitable hassles and adjustments in other domains. Second marriages can be complicated, especially during the initial years. Issues involving stepchildren, the ex-spouse, and in-laws make blended families complex and challenging. An intimate sexual relationship is a solid basis for the marriage and provides motivation to deal with other issues.

Bob and Gloria

One of Barry's most difficult cases involved a couple who were engaged in a power struggle concerning the role of sex in the marriage. Bob was convinced sexual problems had wrecked his first marriage, and was determined that in this marriage sex would be uninhibited and exciting. He insisted Gloria's sexual withholding was the problem. He'd read a number of sex books, attended sexuality workshops, and was committed to putting in the time and energy needed to make this marriage sexually satisfying. Gloria felt on the defensive by Bob's sexual focus, and insisted sex alone would not make their marriage work. Her first marriage, like Bob's, had been a sexual disaster. Gloria attributed this to the husband's immaturity and denial of problems. Sex was only one of a multitude of problems. Gloria felt the only issue Bob was willing to deal with was sexuality, he ignored and avoided talking about other issues and problems. The power struggle centered on Bob's unwillingness to make any agreements about their marriage until sex was spectacular. Gloria was unwilling to deal with sex until Bob showed he cared by taking her to visit friends and relatives, buying a house, and discussing issues affecting their blended family.

Power struggles are counterproductive. They do nothing but build hopelessness and resentment. In a power struggle, not giving in becomes more important than working together to reach marital agreements. You become so caught up in the struggle, you forget what you originally wanted. You are fighting not to

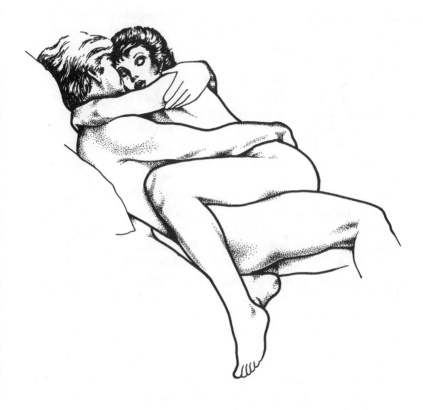

Side-by-side intercourse allows for more connection and communication. Multiple stimulation during intercourse increases eroticism.

win, but to avoid losing. Bob's sexual preoccupation and Gloria's fear of not being respected and cared for caused each to be protective and stubborn.

Barry saw each spouse for five sessions of individual therapy to reduce defensiveness and increase awareness of how self-defeating their stances were. Bob had to recognize there was more to marriage than sex. Gloria realized Bob's reluctance to interact socially with her friends and relatives did not mean he didn't want to be seen with her, but reflected his anxiety that they wouldn't like him. He was afraid he'd be taken advantage of, emotionally or financially, in a marriage where he didn't feel sexually valued. With these issues clarified, they were able to give up their power struggle and move forward.

A major barrier in second marriages is the "fear of a repeat" phenomenon. The spouse is afraid a fight, money problem, sexual dysfunction, or whatever bad experiences caused the first marriage to disintegrate, will recur in this marriage. To prevent that, she avoids fights, does what the other wants, and refuses to discuss hurtful experiences. This avoidance strategy is self-defeating. You have to deal with issues, not avoid them. You can learn from the prior marriage, but cannot let past fears control self-esteem, sexuality and the second marriage. Use awareness as a positive resource, not a rationale for avoidance. Develop a problem-solving approach, working together to deal with sensitive issues.

Mary and George

Mary's first marriage had many problems, but what contributed most to the divorce were fights over money. The husband would become angry and physically abusive. Mary felt incapable of handling money or angry fights.

While she was single again and responsible for money management, she learned to handle finances quite well. In the second marriage, Mary was afraid the money issue and abusive fight pattern would repeat itself. To prevent this, she turned over money, bills, checkbook—all financial matters—to George. She would acquiesce on every issue, doing anything to avoid conflict.

The marriage went reasonably well for the first two years. Then resentments built. George had to assume all financial responsibilities with no help. He was annoyed by Mary's weakness and fear of anything to do with money. He began losing respect for her, and it was not long before loving and sexual feelings also waned. Mary felt George did not make good financial decisions and she did not have enough money to run the household. Constantly trying to avoid arguments caused tension, resulting in headaches. Feelings of competence and confidence she'd developed while single dissipated.

Not working together as a couple spilled over to the sexual area. Sex was routine and infrequent, neither felt a sense of sharing. Resentment from other areas indirectly affects one's sexual relationship. This cycle built on itself and became increasingly corrosive.

Avoiding issues that caused problems in one's first marriage is unrealistic. A more productive strategy is to be aware of and monitor sensitive areas. For example, Mary would tell George that money problems and arguing about them was a trap for her, they needed to work out satisfactory agreements about financial matters. They could develop a plan assigning specific money management responsibilities, and set a monthly time to discuss how the system was working. They would express negative feelings in a nondestructive manner and engage in problem solving to reach agreements instead of fearing destructive, painful fights. After a disagreement, the next day Mary and George would discuss how it was handled, especially whether Mary found it worthwhile to air her feelings, and make sure the resolution was acceptable to both. In marriage, as in other areas of life, a preventive approach is the most efficient and effective. Developing a system to deal with difficult issues and setting aside time to discuss how you're handling them is an excellent strategy to deal with the "avoidance trap."

CLOSING THOUGHTS

Second marriages contain a myriad of practical and emotional issues, including dealing with stepchildren, child support payments, friends and relatives from the prior marriage, feelings of resentment and/or competition regarding the ex-spouse, and functioning as a blended family. Be aware of these issues and be willing to devote time and psychological energy to addressing them. Usually, there is no perfect resolution, but be sure you keep an ongoing dialogue about issues so resentments do not build and carry over to the sexual domain.

Whole books have been written on blended families (stepfamilies). Accept that this family system is different from, and more complex than, the traditional nuclear family. These complexities need to be addressed instead of pretending that everyone loves each other and it's the best possible outcome for all concerned. There are always ambivalent feelings. Some issues will not be resolved—sometimes a child does not like her stepparent, or the ex-spouse continues to be angry and resentful. The best way to deal with these inevitable conflicts and disappointments is to strengthen the primary relationship in the family, the husband-wife bond. Strive to achieve positive changes while accepting that some problems cannot be resolved. Remember, *The Waltons* made great TV, but no family, nuclear or blended, lives up to that ideal.

We would like to reiterate two themes. Learning from the mistakes and problems of one's first marriage greatly increases the probability that you will choose better and the second marriage will be intimate and secure. Second, adopting an open attitude that stresses the need to learn about each other, to communicate feelings and requests, deal with conflict, reach satisfactory agreements, have fun, and develop your sexual style, insures this marriage will be fulfilling and stable.

19
COPING WITH STRESS AND ILLNESS

Our theme throughout this book has been positive: your marital and sexual relationship can be satisfying rather than stagnant and problematic. You continue to learn and grow as individuals and a couple, resulting in enhanced intimacy and satisfaction.

In this chapter, we focus on a reality which has been given only passing attention by marriage and sex books. The sign of a good marriage is not that the couple is happy when external events go well. A vital, solid marriage is demonstrated by the couple's ability to support each other through problems, crisis, illness, and loss. The ability to cope with problems and resolve conflicts is a major marital resource. Some couples naively hope that if they follow our guidelines there will be no marital or sexual difficulties. Nothing could be further from the truth. The more you understand your marital and sexual relationship, the easier it is to prevent falling into common traps. You deal with problems as they arise. Expecting a problem-free relationship is unrealistic, setting you up for frustration and disappointment.

You will be confronted with difficult and disappointing situations. This happens in our lives and marriages, and will in yours. Problems include a parent becoming disabled and needing care, being unemployed for six months, a child with diabetes who needs careful monitoring, your best friends getting divorced, the spouse having colon cancer, an adolescent becoming pregnant, a career risk backfiring, a prostate operation resulting in retrograde ejaculation, a life-threatening accident, an advanced degree or training program doesn't lead to a suitable job, an extramarital affair causing distrust and anger, a job change which necessitates a geographic move causing family disruption. Events such as these can and do happen in most marriages. Some can be prevented, many cannot.

One test of marital viability is the partners' willingness to deal with painful situations. An essential difference between those who maintain psychological well-being and troubled people is not the number of good things that happen, but their ability to cope with stress, conflict, and loss. Coping with difficulties means accepting the reality and regaining equilibrium without major psychological scars. The best way to deal with a crisis is to see it as a challenge and opportunity for learning. If you successfully cope and trust in your spouse, your marriage will be stronger.

Mental health professionals have developed a theory of how people cope with negative experiences and loss, including death. In the first stage there is denial or rejection of the event (it can't be happening). This is followed by a sense of anger (why the hell did this happen to me?) and then a feeling of despair and depression (this is too terrible; I can't deal with it; I'll never be able to accept it). In the final stage, integration, the process reaches a resolution (it was a terrible experience, but we've dealt with it and can go on with our lives). You accept the incident and see yourself as an active survivor rather than a passive victim. Be aware of this process, stay with it, don't repress feelings. You can cope and survive. One of our favorite adages is "Living well is the best revenge." As you reestablish your life and marriage, look back on the stress, illness, or trauma and acknowledge you survived and are back in control. The marriage is psychologically hardy and resilient. Life is meant to be lived in the present, planning for and anticipating the future. It is not meant to be controlled by sadness and resentment from the past.

Jim and Tina

Jim and Tina, a couple in their early forties, had secured a high level of satisfaction. They'd been married seventeen years, had a son fourteen years of age and a daughter of twelve. Jim was an airplane mechanic and Tina an advertising account executive. With two good incomes they lived well, traveled, and engaged in a variety of couple and family activities. They had a good marriage and a vital sexual relationship.

The initial stress came from Tina discovering a lump during a monthly breast self-examination. Her battle with cancer was prolonged. This was physically, financially, and psychologically draining for her, the marriage, and the family. She underwent a mastectomy and extensive chemotherapy. During this time the children were going through adolescence, a stressful time for many families. Jim was afraid of being a widower with two teenagers. His fear made it difficult to listen and emotionally support Tina.

Unlike crises described in books and popular articles, which are intense but limited to hours or days, theirs extended over five years. Tina won her battle with cancer, but, as with all diseases in remission, fears of recurrence continued. Interestingly, they sought marital therapy not during the height of the crisis, but waited until a year had passed (we strongly recommend that couples going through a stressful period seek professional help *at the time*). Both Jim and Tina felt emotionally drained, and their marriage was exhausted. They had sex less than once a month and it was unsatisfying.

They finally stopped avoiding and confronted the reality of their lives and marriage. They began dealing with psychological and relationship issues. The rebuilding process was slow, with several missteps and frustrations, yet they maintained motivation and trust in their marital bond. One of the worst traps was looking back to earlier times, when life seemed natural and simple. Revitalizing the marriage was difficult. They had to overcome inertia. It was difficult setting aside couple time. Jim and Tina had to accept that they were not a young, energetic couple filled with the ecstasy of romantic love, but a middle-years couple who had experienced and coped with a great deal of stress. They needed to reenergize themselves and their marital bond. They couldn't go back to easier times, but had to persevere in recovering from a prolonged crisis and build a satisfying future. They took pride in being a resilient couple, where touching and sexuality once again nurtured their marital bond.

June and Paul

Dealing with loss puts special stress on a marriage. The most painful loss is the death of a child. There is no "right" way to deal with these feelings. It is traumatic and will have a profound effect on you, the marriage, and your sexuality.

Barry began therapy with June and Paul when their son, Ronald, was still in a coma. This eight-year-old boy had suffered severe injuries in a car accident. If he had lived, he would have been profoundly handicapped, physically and intellectually. Therapy sessions sometimes included the entire family, other times just the couple. Individual sessions were scheduled with June who had been driving the car.

The first task was to help them accept the reality of Ronald's impending death. Paul wanted to consult the world's greatest brain surgeon instead of allowing himself to cry and begin grieving the loss of his only son. Ronald's sisters expressed feelings of grief and sadness better than the parents. At the funeral, the minister's sensitive sermon and their friends' genuine sorrow provided support for the family.

In the ensuing months, Paul and June experienced a range of emotions from guilt and anger to listlessness and depression. Gradually they became reinvolved in their lives and experienced times of joy and excitement. They attended to the needs of their daughters, but did not put pressure on them to compensate for the loss of Ronald. They would always consider themselves the parents of three children, one of whom tragically died at age eight. The stress and sadness of that experience did not destroy their marital bond, because June and Paul supported each other through the grieving process. Their sense of trust and being a couple helped them and their children reinvolve themselves in life.

STRESSES OF PARENTING

Parenting is one of the major joys of life. It is also one of the major stresses. This is true of all marriages with children. An ill child or an acting-out or rejecting adolescent can strain the best of marital bonds.

There are two guidelines in understanding and coping with the stresses of parenting. The first is to view the problem in terms of the family system rather than to blame yourself or the child, feel guilty, or give up. The second is to remember that you are first a person, then a spouse, and then a parent. In the long run you will be a better parent if you do not sacrifice your sense of self or marital bond.

Parenting is a crucial role that requires a large and consistent expenditure of time and psychological energy. Celebrate the joys and satisfactions of parenting, but also develop individual and couple activities to provide a respite and reinforcement for parenting. Acknowledge that problems exist rather than pretend everything is perfect. You are not a bad person or a bad mother if you find parenting stressful.

The stress that comes with having a baby can be overwhelming. The fact that a baby is so helpless and needy, combined with lack of skill and worry that you are not the "perfect" caretaker, is draining. When our youngest son was ten days old he stopped breathing. Luckily, our next-door neighbor was an emergency room nurse and revived him. We didn't sleep through the night for several weeks after that incident. During this period, sex was the furthest thing from our minds.

As the child becomes a toddler, you worry he may hurt himself as he explores the world. Many women find the preschool years particularly stressful. You don't have a second to yourself. There is always the possibility of tears or problems. Unless you make specific arrangements and plans, the only time you have to be sexual is late at night when the children are asleep. Late-night sex when you're exhausted is unlikely to promote a creative, playful milieu.

Parents look forward to having more time when children enter school and are surprised to discover new stresses in dealing with teachers, other parents, athletic teams, PTA, etc. Others are sharing the caretaking of your child, but this requires sharing control of the child as well as assuming additional responsibilities. Who will go to parent-teacher meetings, monitor homework, drive car pools? If both parents work, who assumes child care during school holidays, snow days, or illness? Unless you have to deal with these situations, it is hard to describe how difficult and burdensome they can be.

From seven to eleven are the "golden years of childhood." They were among our favorite years of parenting, but this doesn't mean they are stress-free. Trouble with school performance, a difficult adjustment to a friend's moving away, problems with a sibling or neighbor, illness or accident, embarrassment over menstruation or wet dreams—the parent must deal seriously with these concerns rather than treating them lightly or shrugging them off. These experiences matter to the child, and it matters whether you are a caring and responsive parent. Throughout childhood, but especially at this age, it is crucial that you are an "askable parent." The child needs to know she can come to you with questions and psychological and sexual concerns, as well as practical, social and educational matters. A particular problem for children is feeling when something bad happens they need to keep it secret rather than consult the parent as a resource. Each parent needs to both nurture and discipline.

Junior high school (entering adolescence) can be particularly stressful. For many, this is the beginning of experimentation— or at least flirtation—with smoking, drinking, drugs, and sexuality. There is a struggle between peer group and family influence. Children who were good students in elementary school can find the transition to junior high disruptive. Some experience a dramatic drop in academic motivation, and adopt the stance of the alienated adolescent. The type of discipline and rewards that were successful a year before no longer work. The parent who was a "Super Mom" or "Super Dad" two years ago is now a subject of derision for not being "with it."

Are the adolescent years as bad as some say? Certainly not for all adolescents and parents. Thirteen to sixteen is the most unhappy time in a person's life, and for a significant number of parents it's a stressful time in their lives and marriage. The parents' motivation is fear—of pregnancy, drinking and driving, peer pressure, STDs and HIV/AIDS, drugs, self-destructive behavior. Our coping techniques when parenting adolescents were going for walks and out to eat (a positive side effect was that we developed a love of ethnic foods). Emily remembers Barry telling her, "We will survive this and remain a vital couple." There were times when she wondered. In fact, all of us survived. Life gets better after adolescence, not only for the adolescent but for the couple, too.

Parenting does not end when he becomes an eighteen-year-old young adult. It doesn't even end when the person is a twenty-five-year-old adult, even if she is married with children of her own. Parenting becomes less stressful as you take a consultant role and feel less burdened and responsible. That is not always true, especially if you are paying for a child's training program, college, or helping her finance a house. Hopefully, you experience satisfaction from these endeavors.

Much has been written about the "empty nest" phase. Contrary to the cultural myth, the majority of couples report this as a time of increased personal freedom, couple intimacy, and high-quality sex. Couples enjoy parenting, but it's exciting to return to being a couple again and experience a life of reduced stress and responsibility. Sexual satisfaction returns to the high levels you experienced before the birth of the first child.

CHANGING OLD ATTITUDES AND HABITS

Some couples are so strongly tied to old attitudes and habits, they believe change is impossible. They feel the only way out is an affair and/or divorce. You negate the spouse's ability to change and don't believe you can influence her. We knew a man who for twenty-two years bristled because his wife would not leave a party early, afraid she would hurt the hostess's feelings. He felt he could do nothing about this pattern. He did not believe she would listen to a direct request for change, and felt they would never be able to reach a mutually acceptable solution. It is stressful and depressing to feel you are caught in an unsatisfying, unchangeable pattern. A major trap is losing confidence in your ability to make requests, negotiate, and reach an agreement that meets your needs and the needs of the marriage. In a caring relationship, there is always room for change. A friend talked to the wife and made her aware of the husband's frustration. She was open to change and willing to leave parties at a mutually agreeable time. She had not realized how upset he was by this behavior. The husband was surprised and very pleased. She was irritated that he'd sent an emissary rather than talking to her directly.

Ideally, marriage is based on a positive influence process in which you bring out the best in each other. For many couples, the spouse is their best friend, someone to trust, who is honest and not disparaging. As the TV commercials say, it's bad if "even your best friend won't tell you."

We all have idiosyncrasies that were acceptable and, at times, funny when we were younger. As we age, these traits become exaggerated, or we develop habits that are unacceptable to the spouse and others. He has every right to make you aware of this and have enough influence that you attend to the complaint and request for change. The spouse whose drinking is out of control, complains constantly about past job or financial setbacks, has a pattern of watching TV and ignoring family members, gains weight and does not attend to personal appearance, does not keep up couple friendships, or becomes so involved in community and political affairs that marital and family needs are ignored, creates stress. This needs to be confronted. In dating and early marriage, the spouse had a good deal of influence because you wanted him to love and care about you. There is no reason for this to lessen because you're married. In fact, in good marriages, positive influence increases. You are open to share all aspects of your life, including stresses and problems. Value the caring of the spouse and be receptive to her requests.

Jon and Judy

Jon and Judy had a big party to celebrate their silver (twenty-fifth) anniversary. Judy was feeling satisfied with life. She enjoyed the freedom of no children living at home and savored a sense of accomplishment from her job. She was taken aback when, a week after the party, Jon expressed a need to discuss a major problem. He was frustrated with his job and their lifestyle. Years ago, they had moved to the suburbs because they wanted a larger home and better schools. It had been an excellent environment in which to raise children. Now, Jon wanted to move to a townhouse in the city, both to reduce commuting time and take advantage of the restaurants and cultural offerings of the city. He wanted to resign and set up his own consulting firm so he could implement creative ideas. Judy was distressed because she identified with her home and neighborhood. Her job was in a shopping mall less than a mile away.

A key element in marriage is the ability to state individual needs and feelings. Jon had done that very well. Clear and direct communication is important in marriage, but does not automatically make things all right. It took a great deal of discussion and negotiation, considering both practical and psychological aspects, before a mutually acceptable agreement was reached.

They moved to a townhouse in an area of the city that Judy enjoyed. She became involved in the new community but retained her job in the suburbs and bought a sports car she could enjoy commuting in. Jon kept a consulting position with his employer rather than starting completely on his own. These decisions reflect the practical components of the agreement.

More important was discussion of the psychological and relationship-related meanings of the change. Instead of allowing their good marriage to "go along as is," Jon and Judy made a renewed commitment to individual and couple growth. Jon knew a number of friends who were dissatisfied with their jobs, marriages, and sex lives. He saw them drinking too much, having heart attacks, starting affairs with twenty-five-year-old secretaries, and becoming cynical and depressed. He was determined this would not happen to him or the marriage. Judy was able to hear Jon's feelings, anxieties, and requests without becoming fearful or defensive. One of their marital strengths was a sense of trust and equity. This allowed Judy to frankly discuss her desires, feelings, and anxieties. She would not give in to Jon out of weakness or agree to something she couldn't live with. Judy knew what was important to her, and was able to state that. From a position of awareness and caring, they discussed feelings and realistic alternatives. Jon and Judy negotiated an agreement both could live with and that would enhance the next phase of their lives.

A key element of a vital marriage is openness to change and growth. The traditional assumption was that marriage is characterized by stability. Although stability and security are important, so are change and growth. People's lives, jobs, and parenting roles experience transitions. This includes changes in sexual desire and functioning. The basis of creative sexuality is an integration of the familiar and the secure (what you've learned brings sexual pleasure) and the immediate moods, techniques, and desires you bring to each encounter. Your sexual relationship remains alive and vital because of openness to change and new experiences. Marital trust and security provides the solid basis that allows you to be spontaneous and experimental, to take risks and be sexually creative. Intimacy and sexuality energize your marital bond and make it special.

SEXUAL STRESS

One of the best-kept secrets is that the great majority of couples undergo a period of sexual stress sometime in their marriage. This can be caused by a specific sexual problem, such as erectile dysfunction, inhibited sexual desire, or painful intercourse; by a marital or family problem such as financial stress, a child in trouble, or a falling-out with in-laws; by an individual problem such as depression, overwork, a strained back; or by an unexplained sense of malaise. How can a couple cope with sexual stress? Admit this period is problematic and unhappy, but do not panic or overreact. Accept the spouse and maintain affectionate and sensual contact. Especially when sex is in remission, caring, affection, and sensuality need to be nurtured and expressed. This atmosphere of acceptance without blame allows a smoother return to satisfying sex as the issue is dealt with and the stress dissipates.

Some bemoan the loss of ecstasy in marital sex. If you examine ecstasy, you find it in premarital and extramarital affairs. The elements that comprise passion and ecstasy are novelty, overcoming frustrations and barriers in order to be with the partner, unpredictability, desire to be accepted and/or win the partner, and a sense of illicitness. This adventuresome, romantic notion of love is by definition fragile and temporary. It can and should be replaced by a mature sense of caring, security, respect, trust, and intimacy. This provides a solid basis for a satisfying, stable marriage. Intimacy and sexuality helps you through the inevitable stresses human beings and relationships encounter.

EPILOGUE
IS THERE SEX AFTER MARRIAGE?

This completes a four-book sequence. The first book, *Sexual Awareness* focused on specific exercises to improve sexual comfort, pleasure and functioning. *Male Sexual Awareness* and *Female Sexual Awareness* focused on changing sexual attitudes, behavior, and emotional responsiveness. *Couple Sexual Awareness* is the crown jewel of the series. Optimal sexual functioning integrates intimacy and sexuality in the context of a secure marital bond.

Both women and men can be comfortable and skilled at sexual initiation, sharing intimate feelings, nondemand pleasuring, eroticism, being orgasmic, and feeling satisfied and bonded. Sex is more than genitals, intercourse, and orgasm. Sexuality is a positive, integral component of the marital bond. It serves as a shared pleasure, a way to maintain and reinforce intimacy, and a tension reducer to deal with the stresses of life and the marriage. When sexuality is going well, it is fifteen to twenty percent of the relationship, its primary function being to energize the marital bond.

We have presented guidelines, strategies, and techniques to increase marital and sexual satisfaction. Each couple develops their unique marital and sexual style. We urge you to value the marriage and devote time and psychological energy to nurture your marital bond. However, we are not romantic idealists. There are no perfect people, no perfect jobs, no perfect children, no perfect houses, and no perfect marriages. Romantic images of marriage need to be replaced by positive, realistic expectations and mature intimacy. The marital bond of respect and trust enables you to accept your spouse and marriage for its strengths and joys as well as vulnerabilities and problems. Marriage and marital sex are not static, they involve a process of change and growth. Marriage works best when it is based on a positive influence model. That kind of marriage brings out the best in you.

Sexuality can be a satisfying part of life and marriage. The essence of sexuality is giving and receiving pleasure-oriented touch. Sexuality functions best in the context of a respectful, trusting, emotionally intimate marriage based on a sense of equity between the woman and man. You owe it to yourself, your spouse, and family to devote the time and psychological energy to make your marriage and marital sex satisfying and stable.

APPENDIX I
CHOOSING A THERAPIST

As stated in the first chapter, this is not a do-it-yourself therapy book. Couples are reluctant to consult a therapist, feeling to do so is a sign of "craziness," inadequacy, or that their marriage is in dire straits and about to end. In reality, seeking professional help is a sign of psychological strength. Entering marital or sex therapy means you realize there is a problem and have made a commitment to resolving the issues and promoting marital and sexual growth.

The mental health field can be confusing. Marital and sex therapy are clinical subspecialties. They are offered by several groups of professionals, including psychologists, social workers, marriage therapists, psychiatrists, sex therapists, and pastoral counselors. The professional background of the practitioner is of less importance than her competency in dealing with your specific problem.

Many people have health insurance that provides coverage for mental health, and thus can afford the services of a private practitioner. Those who do not have either financial resources or insurance could consider a city or county mental health clinic, a university or medical school mental health outpatient clinic or a family services center. Clinics usually have a sliding fee scale. The fee is based on your ability to pay.

In choosing a therapist, be assertive in asking about credentials and areas of expertise. Ask the clinician what percentage of her clients stay married, how long the therapy can be expected to last, and whether there is a specific focus on communication, problem solving, and/or sexual problems. A competent therapist will be open to discussing these issues. Be especially diligent in questioning credentials such as university degrees and licensing of people who call themselves personal counselors, marriage counselors, or sex counselors. There are poorly qualified persons—and some outright quacks—in any field.

One of the best resources for obtaining a referral is to call a local professional organization such as a psychological association, marriage and family therapy association, mental health association, or mental health clinic. You can ask for a referral from a family physician, minister, or friend. If you are specifically interested in sex therapy, you can write the American Association of Sex Educators, Counselors, and Therapists, P.O. Box 238, Mount Vernon, IA 52314, (319) 895-8407, for a list of certified sex therapists in your area.

Feel free to talk with two or three therapists before deciding on one with whom to work. Be aware of comfort with the therapist, degree of rapport, and whether the therapist's assessment of the problem and approach to treatment make sense to you. Once you begin, give therapy a chance to be helpful. There are few miracle cures. Change requires commitment and is a gradual and often difficult process. Although some couples benefit from short-term therapy (fewer than ten sessions), most couples find the therapeutic process will take four months to a year or longer. The role of the therapist is that of a consultant rather than decision maker. Therapy requires effort, both in the session and at home. Therapy focuses on changing attitudes, feelings, and behavior, making your marital and sexual life more satisfying.

APPENDIX II
BOOKS FOR FURTHER READING

Andry, Andrew and Steve Schepp. *How Babies Are Made*. Boston: Little, Brown, 1984.

Bing, Elizabeth and Libby Coleman. *Making Love during Pregnancy*. New York: Bantam Books, 1983.

Butler, Robert and Myrna Lewis. *Love and Sex after Sixty*. New York: Ballantine, 1993.

Castleman, Michael. *Sexual Solutions*. New York: Simon and Schuster, 1989.

Gordon, Sol. *Why Love Is Not Enough*. Boston: Bob Adams, 1990.

Gottman, John. *Why Marriages Succeed or Fail*. New York: Simon and Schuster, 1994.

Heiman, Julia and Joseph LoPiccolo. *Becoming Orgasmic*. New York: Prentice Hall, 1988.

Lehner, Harriet. *The Dance of Anger*. New York: Harper and Row, 1985.

Leight, Lynn. *Raising Sexually Healthy Children*. New York: Avon, 1990.

Maltz, Wendy. *The Sexual Healing Journey*. New York: HarperCollins, 1991.

McCarthy, Barry and Emily McCarthy. *Male Sexual Awareness*. New York: Carroll and Graf, 1998.

———. *Sexual Awareness*. New York: Carroll & Graf, 1993.

———. *Female Sexual Awareness*. New York: Carroll & Graf, 1989.

———. *Intimate Marriage*. New York: Carroll & Graf, 1992.

———. *Confronting the Victim Role.* New York: Carroll & Graf, 1993.

Michael, Robert, John Gagnon, Edward Laumann, and Gina Kolota. *Sex in America.* Boston: Little, Brown, 1994.

Moglia, Ronald and Jon Knowles. *All about Sex: A Family Resource on Sex and Sexuality.* Westminster, MD: Random House, 1997.

Notarius, Cliff and Howard Markman. *We Can Work It Out.* New York: Putnam, 1993.

Trafford, Abigail. *Crazy Time: Surviving Divorce and Building a New Life.* New York: Harper Perennial, 1992.

Zilbergeld, Bernie. *New Male Sexuality.* New York: Bantam Books, 1992.

Zoldbrod, Aline. *Sex Smart.* Oakland: New Harbinger, 1998.